Praise for *Healing Animals*

DR MICHAEL W FOX is a national treasure. In his latest book he moves through a wide scope of worldwide plight of animals wild and domestic. He allows his readers inside his heart and mind, and this is the heart of a healer in every sense of the word. They will smile in remembrance, cry is sympathy and share anger at things unjust, but mostly they will awaken their inner voices and hopefully listen more to that Truth that resides in every sentient Being, for it is that which makes us civilized, happy and truly prosperous.
RICHARD PALMQUIST, DVM, Chief of Integrative Veterinary Health Services, Centinela Animal Hospital, President-elect and research chair, AHVMA
Author of *Integrating Complementary Medicine into Veterinary Practice*

Healing Animals will rock your conceptual world. It is the end all be all Book … no further reading is required for an instant shift in ones consciousness with regards to how animals and the earth are viewed, experienced and treated. It is a must read for all veterinarians, healers and animal care givers.
DR. BOB AND SUSAN GOLDSTEIN, Authors of *The Wellness and Longevity Program for Dogs and Cats*

After almost two decades practicing veterinary medicine, I am still learning how to muscle through times of despair, those days I lose more lives than I save, and Dr. Fox's new book, *Healing Animals*, will help to fortify the healer within all of us. Dr. Fox uses research and his unique perspective working in developing countries to point out numerous ethical dilemmas facing our profession: Overdependence on corporate profit margins has eroded quality animal husbandry and compassionate care. Through this book, we learn the problems of agribusiness, vaccination, and commercial pet and livestock food as well as solutions, such as consuming less meat, control of genetically modified food and the importance of eating organic. Thank you Dr Fox for injecting a bit of hybrid vigor into our practices and reminding us that we will always have the most important aspect of being compassionate veterinarians—our ability to discern and dissect the truth and keep a critical eye on the origin of information.
DONNA KELLEHER, DVM, Author of *The Last Chance Dog*

Dr. Michael Fox has done it again. Dr. Fox has always been a role model for me, both as an animal behaviorist and a pioneer in holistic, integrative veterinary medicine. His new book is a pinnacle of his career. He dares to speak the truth about human animal relations and its implications for the 21st century. Kudos to Dr. Fox for sharing his wisdom and insights in a heartfelt, professional book that will touch animal lovers and stimulate them to action throughout the world.
Allen M. Schoen, MS, DVM, Author of *Kindred Spirits*

As I read this book I found remarkable parallels with my own life – like Michael Fox I loved ponds when a child (and almost drowned in one). I also had a burning desire to work with animals. I too trained at the Royal Veterinary College, London, and, like Michael, I left conventional veterinary medicine to pursue a different veterinary track. In my case it was to specialize in natural therapies such as homeopathy and acupuncture. In Michael's case, it has been a career of work with animal protection and welfare.

This book is a distillation of his lifetime's work with animals. Dr. Fox reveals the suffering animals endure at the hand of humans, explains the interconnectedness of humans and animals with each other and with the world itself, and details the many ways in which science and agribusiness is causing damage and destruction to farm animals and crops, to pets, to humans and to the earth itself.

It is a thought provoking book, one which will make anyone who reads it more aware of the existing and potential risks to us, our animals and our environment, and the need to take action before it is too late.

RICHARD ALLPORT, BVetMed, VetMFHom, MRCVS
The Natural Medicine Centre, Potters Bar, Herts, England

I have had the pleasure of knowing the author for several decades as we've traversed parallel yet different paths focused on the health and well-being of all sentient beings. We both graduated within two years of each other, Michael in the UK, myself in Canada.

This manuscript is heartfelt and offers important yet painful sorties into the myriad complexities of our "modern" world. It is a cautionary tale, which charts our path through the choppy waters of commercialism, commoditization, and exploitation on the world platform. Some would call this progressive, others see it as a disaster in the making.

The first important message of this manuscript is: "Human Well-being means Health Care People Care + Animal Care + Earth Care." Following that comes discussion and ranking of animal suffering worldwide. Powerful words follow in "those qualities or virtues that makes us human – humility, compassion and selfless benevolence—will continue to be crushed by the arrogance, ignorance and selfishness of our species." Next we have "reducing animal consumption: a bioethical imperative," as "The singularly most damaging environmental footprint upon this planet is caused by our collectively costly and damaging appetite for meat." He further states that "The incorporation of cloned and transgenic farm animals into conventional, industrial agriculture is ethically, economically and environmentally unacceptable." Chapters addressing conflicts in the veterinary profession, the tripartite nature of holistic medicine, the genetic engineering and cloning of animals, and documented concerns about many manufactured pet foods are exceptionally compelling. Bravo, my friend!

W. JEAN DODDS, DVM
Hemopet/Hemolife, Garden Grove CA

BOOKS BY DR. MICHAEL W. FOX

Not Fit for a Dog: The Truth about Manufactured Dog and Cat Food, co-authored with Elizabeth Hodgkins, DVM, Esq, and Marion E. Smart, DVM, PhD, Sanger CA, Quill Driver Books, 2008

Dog Body, Dog Mind: Exploring Canine Consciousness and Total Well-Being. Guilford, CT. The Lyon's Press, 2007

Cat Body, Cat Mind: Exploring Feline Consciousness and Total Well-Being. Guilford, CT. The Lyons Press, 2007

Bring Life to Ethics: Global Bioethics for a Humane Society. Albany, NY, State University of New York Press, 2001

Killer Foods: When Scientists Manipulate Genes, Better is Not Always Best. Guilford, CT. The Lyons Press, 2004

The Healing Touch for Dogs. New York: Newmarket Press, 2004

The Healing Touch for Cats. New York: Newmarket Press, 2004

Eating with Conscience: The Bioethics of Food. Troutdale, Oregon: New Sage Press, 1997

Concepts in Ethology, Animal Behavior and Bioethics (revised edition). Malabar, FL: R. E. Krieger Publishing Co., 1997

The Boundless Circle. (1996) Quest Books, Wheaton, Illinois

Supercat. New York, NY, Howell Books, 1991.

The New Eden. (1989) Lotus Press, Santa Fe, New Mexico 1989

The New Animal Doctor's Answer Book. Newmarket Press, New York 1989

Laboratory Animal Husbandry. State University of New York Press, Albany, New York 1986

The Whistling Hunters. State University of New York Press, Albany, New York 1984

Love is a Happy Cat. Newmarket Press, New York 1982

Out of print (Available on amazon.com, alibris.com, abebooks.com)

Agricide: The Hidden Farm and Food Crisis that Affects Us All (revised edition 1996) R.E. Krieger Publishing Co., Malabar, Florida, 1996.

The Soul of the Wolf. (reprint edition 1992) Lyons & Burford, New York

Understanding Your Dog. (revised edition 1992) St. Martin's Press, New York

Understanding Your Cat. (revised edition 1992) St. Martin's Press, New York

You Can Save the Animals. (1991) St. Martin's Press, New York

Superdog. (1990) Howell Books, New York

Inhumane Society: The American Way of Exploiting Animals. (1990) St Martin's Press, NY

Between Animal and Man: The Key to the Kingdom. (reprint edition 1986) Krieger Publishing Co., Malabar, Florida

Behavior of Wolves, Dogs, and related Canids (reprint edition1984). Krieger Publishing Co., Malabar, Florida

One Earth, One Mind (reprint edition 1984) Krieger Publishing Co., Malabar, Florida

Farm Animals: Husbandry, Behavior and Veterinary Practice. (1983) University Press, Baltimore, Maryland

How to be Your Pet's best Friend (1981) Coward, McCann & Geoghegan, New York.

Returning to Eden: Animal Rights and Human responsibility (1980) Viking Press, New York
Understanding Your Pet (1978) Coward, McCann and Geoghegan, New York
Canine Behavior (reprint edition 1972) Charles C. Thomas Publishing, Springfield, Illinois
Integrative Development of Brain and Behavior in the Dog (1971) University of Chicago Press
Canine Pediatrics (1966) Charles C. Thomas Publishing, Springfield, Illinois

Editor of

Advances in Animal Welfare Science (annual series 1984-1987) Martinus Nijhoff in Holland, and The Humane Society of the United States, Washington, DC
The Dog: Its Domestication and Behavior. (reprint edition 1987) Krieger Publishing Co., Malabar, Florida
The Wild Canids (reprint edition 2009) DogWise Books, www.dogwise.com
On the Fifth day: Animal Rights and Human Ethics (1977) Acropolis Press, Washington, DC (With R. K. Morris)
Readings in Ethology and Comparative Psychology. (1973) Brooks/Cole, California
Abnormal Behavior in Animals. (1968) Saunders, Philadelphia

Children's Books

Animals Have Rights Too (1991) Crossroads/Continuum, New York
The Way of the Dolphin (1981) Acropolis Books, Washington, DC
The Touchlings (1981) Acropolis Books, Washington, DC
Lessons from Nature: Fox's Fables (1980) Acropolis, Washington, DC
Whitepaws: A Coyote Dog (1979) Coward, McCann & Geoghegan, New York
Wild Dogs Three (1977) Coward, McCann & Geoghegan, New York
What is Your Dog Saying? (1977) M. W. Fox and Wende Devlin Gates, Coward, McCann & Geoghegan, New York
What is Your Cat Saying? (1977) M. W. Fox and Wende Devlin Gates, Coward, McCann & Geoghegan, New York
*Ramu and Chennai** (1975) Coward, McCann & Geoghegan, New York
*Sundance Coyote^* (1974) Coward, McCann & Geoghegan, New York
The Wolf~ (1973) Coward, McCann & Geoghegan, New York
Vixie, The Story of a Little Fox (1973) Coward, McCann & Geoghegan, New York

*   Best Science Book Award, National Teachers' Association
^   Nominee for Mark Twain Award
~   Christopher Award for children's literature

Healing Animals
&
The Vision of One Health

Earth Care and Human Care

A Veterinary Testimony & a Personal Testament

By Dr. Michael W. Fox

Foreword by Dr. Steve Marsden

One Health Vision Press

Sarasota

Cover Photograph: 2011, M.W. Fox. One of several vultures found dying from eating poisoned bait put out to kill livestock predators in the Nilgiri Biosphere Reserve, South India
Author photograph: Deanna Krantz
Graphics: M.W. Fox and as noted

Published by One Health Vision Press,
M&RW Ltd, at SynGeo ArchiGraph
    8051 North Tamiami Trail, No. 70
    Post Office Box 370
    Tallevast, Florida 34270

For more information on sites and projects
or to contact the author:
    Two Bit Dog: www.twobitdog.com/drfox/
    SynGeo ArchiGraph LLC: www.syngeo.org

Publisher's Cataloging in Publication Data
Michael W. Fox 1937—
Healing Animals & the Vision of One Health / Michael W. Fox
Includes bibliographical references

ISBN 1-461150-28-0
ISBN13 978-1-461150-28-2

1. Veterinary Medicine. 2. Agriculture & Food. 3. Environmental Health
I. Title.

Book Design by Rian Garcia Calusa
    www.riangarciacalusa.com
    M&RW Ltd: www.reasonwolf.com

Printed in the United States of America

CONTENTS

FOR DEANNA KRANTZ
Wife and comrade

FOREWORD

Disillusionment is common in the healing arts. The idealism with which most doctors brim on entering their professions often and sadly becomes replaced with a sense of resignation, as the limits of the theoretical and financial underpinnings of the western medical model become apparent. Therapeutic goals shift from a desire to better the lot of their patient's life, to simply palliating their symptoms and slowing their decline. Career success gets increasingly defined in terms of time off and income, and increasingly less in terms of client and patient satisfaction and well-being. Gradually, inexorably, the humanitarian glands of many practitioners shrivel with age and lack of exercise.

Dr. Michael Fox stands out against this jaded backdrop. He is known worldwide for being a voice of compassion and empathy for animals, and is the idol of countless veterinary students still steeped in idealism. His long career as a veterinarian has not inured him at all to the plight of animals. Quite the opposite, in fact, and he is perhaps most famous for his illumination and extolling of the human-animal bond that is the source of such rich rewards for both pets and their owners.

In his new book, *Healing Animals*, Dr. Fox extends his gaze not only to the pet industry, but animal agriculture and the environment as a whole. The general message is the same, however: The inter-dependent nature of human and animal welfare. While the theme is consistent, the particulars are new. They are also quite alarming.

The title 'Healing Animals', as noted by Dr. Fox, is a double entendre. It implies both the mutual reliance of humans upon animals, and animals upon humans, for their collective well being. As such, then, Animal Healing is a book about wise stewardship.

Regrettably, however, a wide gulf has appeared in the last half century between what we know to be true regarding wise stewardship of animals, and what we actually end up doing for them. The provinces that abut this gulf include more than the usual realms of veterinary medicine and animal agriculture. Animal healing is coming increasingly to rely just as much upon influences as remote and diverse as policies made by government in hallowed halls; choices made by consumers in the grocery line up; subsidies offered to farmers by governments; the insistent demand of shareholders on corporations to increase profits; and the way healthcare is provided and funded by government and insurance corporations.

Dr. Fox explores these interfaces and more to lay out for us the full extent of what exactly they bring to bear on the health and well being of animals. The reader will immediately realize, upon diving into the book, that *Healing Animals* is nothing short of a magnum opus. It is meticulously researched, exploring in unparalleled breadth and depth the medical, agricultural, government, and societal trends, beliefs and policies that impact the natural world and threaten to unwittingly mortgage our future for many generations to come. It offers both a '30,000 foot view' and, at other times, a detailed analysis to illuminate all that is wrong with the way we take care of animals and our environment. It is a book that has never been written before, and which would take an enormous amount of heart to ever write again.

In reading Healing Animals, one cannot help but be struck by the interdependencies and connectedness of our current agricultural, economic, political, healthcare, and eco- systems. There is scarcely a person among us who will not be implicated in its discussion, and who therefore does not hold the fate of some component of the natural world in their grasp. If one lives in an industrial society, the book should be required reading.

Healing Animals is thus an invocation to the collective power of us all to change our systems and values before it is too late. But how to take that first step? Who should take it, and in so doing, lead the rest of us to a brave new world?

In reading the book and becoming aware of the enormous effort needed to improve the lot of animals, the earth and ourselves, it becomes apparent we face no less than the Lernaean Hydra, the multi-headed and seemingly indestructible monster of Greek folklore. As one head was chopped off, two more would grow. The secret to the destruction of the Hydra by Hercules was to find the one head amongst dozens that was the secret of the beast's immortality. Chop this off, and the beast dies.

As you read this book you will naturally seek this crucial weakness of our own Hydra, but perhaps be left believing it is an impossible task. In this web of interconnectedness involving all levels of government and spheres of human endeavour, how can we possibly identify the one problem on which all other factors influencing animal welfare depend? The temptation will be strong to crawl back under a rock and seek solace in ignorance.

Upon further reflection, however, the answer to the Hydra riddle will become obvious. In this monster of our own making, the enduring threat is not capitalism, pollution, or even ignorance. Rather, it is simple human greed—the continual prioritization of our own needs first. Ironically, then, considering the convoluted nature of the mutual problems that face both us and our animal friends, we need no leader to take the initiative. Overpowering the instinctive pursuit of self-interest in each of us is all that is required to take the first important step, and the power to do so rests with no one but ourselves. After that, we need only a compass bearing, a polestar, to guide us on our way. Dr. Fox has provided that for us in this book.

Dr. Steve Marsden
Alberta, Canada
Named Small Animal Veterinarian of the Year
By the Canadian Veterinary Medical Association, 2009.

INTRODUCTION

As I prepared to go to my fiftieth class reunion at the Royal Veterinary College of London University, England, I found myself reflecting on my career and many endeavors aimed at fulfilling my professional vow to use my skills for the benefit of animals' health and well-being. In the following pages I have laid out some of my experiences and concerns that will interest and inform pet owners and animal lovers in general. I hope to inspire a new generation of veterinarians and other dedicated healers to think 'outside the box' to rectify the declining health of the environment and especially of concentrated animal and human populations around the world.

Animal farmers, caretakers and others involved in various commercial uses of animals will find themselves confronted by the realities and consequences of animal exploitation, and join me in finding humane alternatives and ways to improve animal health and welfare. I have met many good veterinarians as well as agricultural and animal scientists in industry and academia, and have seen many in their ranks move forward in their thinking, even putting their careers at risk in their advocacy for animal welfare and basic rights, and for good ecological stewardship practices by all forms of industry and commerce.

Specialist organizations, both governmental and nongovernmental, have been formed to address these issues, and related environmental and conservation concerns. Through this collection of essays I will show the interconnection among these issues and concerns. Many solutions may lie in a pooling of professional expertise from several specialist disciplines to help solve the local, national and global problems that we face today. But ultimately our health and well-being, and of our loved ones as well as all living beings under our care, including those in various environments we affect directly and indirectly, is a personal responsibility. As I will show, neither science nor God or government can make us well. That is our responsibility and duty when it comes to caring for others in need such as our children and companion and farmed animals.

This makes a book such as this a book for a very wide audience because we all depend in one way or another on animals for food, clothing, companionship, even advances in our own health and spiritual well-being. We all therefore have an ethical obligation to include animals and the environment in the human community of moral concern and legal protection. This ethical mandate begins with us as consumers and pet owners, and ends with government regulatory agencies and industries awakening to the call of bioethics to extend the Golden Rule to the broader life community of which we humans are a small, inter-dependent part.

Through my personal history and professional opinions supported by scientific and clinical reviews, I present my vision of what the future holds for our species and that of the Earth community when we treat nonhuman life with respect and gratitude long overdue. I make no apologies in the sections where I use medical and other scientific terms. To simplify complex issues in layman's language will create a kind of opacity and illiteracy once fostered by the Towers of Babel but now by contemporary institutions and professional organizations, religious and secular. Wherever I use specialist terms I explain their meaning in the text or as a endnote to serve a wider readership.

Healing Animals has a double meaning. Animals will heal us as we heal them by repairing the bond we have with them. This healing entails the recovery of our humanity and our capacity to empathize so deeply with animals that we begin to feel the world through their senses. As we heal our relationship with Nature and animals, a radical revision of the history of our civilization and a redefinition of what it means to be human will occur. We will evaluate what we are doing with our lives and by our actions how we benefit or harm the animal kingdom and the natural, original First World.

My life's goal as a veterinarian and humane advocate is to help establish mutually beneficial relationships between humanity and the animal kingdom. I believe that a primary role for the veterinary profession is to help heal the bond between humans, animals and Nature. This was the role of shamans and healers in other cultures long before ours.

Scientifically, Healing Animals also has a double meaning. Carefully controlled studies have shown that gently handled animals, be they pigs, chickens, rats or rabbits, can increase their resistance to stress and disease. Much of my research on animals in the 1960's and 70's was in this fascinating aspect of the human-animal bond. When a strong bond is established, based on trust, the emotional and physiological responses of animals to their human caretakers or companions contribute positively to the animals' psychological and physical well-being.

When enhanced by our empathy and understanding, the human-animal bond is a reciprocal relationship where animals can heal us. As a consequence of what I call sympathetic resonance, animals can affect us emotionally and physiologically as profoundly and as beneficially, as we can affect them. These discoveries are as significant as those of quantum physics. This, which I see as a "second scientific revolution"— has profound implications in terms of our relationships with animals and Nature and what it means to be human. This second scientific revolution opens up new dimensions — ethical, emotional, metaphysical and spiritual — that mechanistic science and derivative medical and other technologies, by their very nature, exclude. This revolution will have far-reaching, global economic, ecological, social and political consequences. Today these are already evident in new developments in holistic, integrative medicine and organic ecological farming. It is bringing about a paradigm-shift, a change in our worldview, from one that is human-centered or anthropocentric to one that is more Earth or Creation-centered. In the process, we will begin the incredible task of healing the Earth and of healing humanity by restoring the many connections, spiritual and physical, that bind us to the natural world and sustain all

In recounting the events, experiences, and the gifts of creatures both great and small that set my life on this course, readers will find affirmation of their own feelings about animals and Nature. I hope this book will serve as an eye and heart opener for many readers and that they will also join me in healing animals healing us. This is not simply the veterinary profession's task, but everyone's responsibility.

Golden Valley
Minnesota, May 2010

CHAPTER 1
Early Experiences, Enduring Connections

My first encounters with the miraculous and the mysterious were almost daily as a child. I had a playground full of miracles. It included an area called "the jungle" a wasteland thicket full of wild things. But for World War II, it would have been obliterated by the expansion of the suburban housing development where I was raised for the first ten years of my life. There were six ponds scattered close by on half-wild farmland where there were fields of corn, turnips, and pastures for cattle. A meandering public footpath lined with brambles, black and purple with shining berries in the fall that traversed a heath turned into a children's playing field for summer cricket and winter soccer, was my daily way to the ponds, jungle and fields.

Like the child in Walt Whitman's poem who went out into the world and became all that he perceived, I entered the numinous world of Nature that my playground embraced, and felt myself become a part of everything.

The microcosm of a pond is truly awesome in its beauty, subtlety, order and complexity: a universe in miniature and a relatively alien world to us terrestrial talking bipeds. This I recognized and appreciated as a child. To play with a pond — and by that I mean to examine at close hand, to "mind" everything that I perceived in it, on it, and around it — was indeed to experience the miraculous. And each pond was different.

One was the sanctum of the Great Crested Newt; and in another pond lived the water spider who built an underwater net and secured a large bubble of air in it within which her offspring developed and hatched. My least favorite pond was the most scary, with banks so steep the cattle never came to drink, and with its surface covered in a green carpet of floating pond weed.

My first involvement with ponds was before my earliest memories. I was told that I nearly drowned when, under the inattentive eye of a young babysitter, I decided to walk into one of the ponds to pet some dabbling mallard ducks.

But it was no near-death experience that made me cherish and revere the miraculous. It was the life that I discovered in my playground where I invariably played alone from the age of six and on, since none of my peers had much interest in the ponds except in occasionally killing whatever they might catch therein with nets and wiggling worms impaled on bent pins.

The ponds taught me the laws of the universe—that there is a seamless web of life wherein the forces of creation and destruction are in balance, so that everything is contained in a state of harmony, health, and beauty.

Disconnections

The ponds not only taught me about Nature, they also taught me much about human nature. One springtime, when the frogs were mating and could be easily caught when males were clasped around their larger mates, I found over a dozen of them torn to pieces on the bank of the pond. No creature could have done that and left all those frog pieces uneaten. I saw small boot prints only a little bigger than mine in the mud around them, and broken hollow grass stems in the carnage. One piece was still protruding from the mouth of one of the frogs. Its belly had burst open and the entrails were caked in mud. I never understood what had happened to them until some years later I learned that you can blow up a frog until it bursts like a balloon if you blow into a straw shoved down its gullet or in its rectum. Such was the nature of my playmates, most of whom I avoided at the best of times.

The other insight into human nature was no less shocking and was easier for my child mind to realize what had happened. I had just celebrated my seventh birthday and was mucking around the edge of one of the ponds looking to see what creatures I might, when I noticed a large burlap sack floating in the middle of the pond. I went into the "jungle" and broke off the longest elderberry branch I could find, waded into the pond and pulled the sack out. Treasure, I thought: Some robber's loot. I tore the bag open and recoiled in horror. A whole litter of kittens, their eyes unopened and their rotting bodies swollen almost beyond recognition, assailed my senses. I was dumbfounded. How and why could anyone do such a thing to such beautiful little creatures?

More than fifty years after my first experience seeing others deliberately afflicting cruelty on frogs, and I believe they did it for the pure fun of watching frogs burst like little green and yellow balloons, I am still shocked and perplexed by this human proclivity to delight in another's suffering and helplessness. How the frogs must have struggled, with brains still intact but bodies blown apart, and how my peers must have enjoyed the spectacle, laughing and catching more frogs to torture and kill for pleasure.

Why do humans enjoy killing defenseless creatures? Driving to work one morning, I found myself tearing-up, thinking about the book review of the late English writer Lorna Sage's book *Bad Blood: A Memoir* (2002, Morrow: London and New York). The review (*Washington Post* 3/24/2002) by Michael Dirda aptly entitled "Running Wild," included:

Sage meanwhile wanders the fields around her housing complex, idyllically at home in woods and farmland. But local agricultural tradition included some "rackety field sports" straight out of The Golden Bough:

'For instance, each field's crop was cut so as to leave a small plot of corn standing in the middle. Then, when the combine harvester had done thudding, everyone, the labourer's families, kids and hangers-on, would converge on this corn island with hoots and yells, sticks and pitchforks, and murder the mass of voles, mice and rabbits that had taken shelter there as they made a last mad dash for safety.'

Reading this account reminded me of my old friend and animal suffragist Cleveland Amory, who battled the rural 'Bunny Boppers' of rural America and, with others, fought the rattlesnake, prairie dog, and coyote exterminators.

The delight in extermination and witnessing same, for reasons myriad, and consequences prophetically karmic (violence begets violence), is a potentially fatal flaw in the human psyche. We all, with few exceptions, know better, once we understand the connection between the love of Nature and the nature of true love.

What I find particularly chilling is the human capacity to disconnect in a moment – and throughout our recorded history – from feeling for every living being within one's sphere of relationship and immediate presence.

I once felt this chill watching a circle of people beneath a platform lamp at a rural railway station watch a large moth flutter weakly down from the light and continue their animated conversation while they look on as a six or seven-year old girl standing with them rubbed the moth into a silken paste on the platform under one of her dainty shoes.

When I was in sixth grade, I sometimes decided to walk home rather than take the bus. There was a girl called Hilary I hoped to see, since she lived near the school and always walked home, which was along my bus route. My route took me past the local veterinary clinic and on an impulse I went to have a closer look. I saw the animal doctor's polished brass plate by the door with his degree letters after his name:'

M.R.C.V.S.'—Member of the Royal Veterinary College. That's what being "qualified" means, I realized, and that entailed going to a university and years of study, I guessed.

To the left of the door was a window that looked in on his clinic, but being small for my age, I couldn't quite see in. Then I heard a cat meowing from behind a fence at the back of the clinic and I peered through. At first I couldn't understand what I was seeing. There were two metal trash cans filled to the top with dead dogs and cats with a halo of flies buzzing noisily over each. The prowling cat that I had heard ran out of the yard, scaling the fence in one bound. I crouched down, taking in the scene of horror, thinking of the kittens in the sack I had found in the pond and wondering why, and again a great sadness came over me.

I didn't reason that the veterinarian had killed them all because of some epidemic disease, or because people didn't want them or couldn't afford to feed them properly because food was tightly rationed in early post-war England. I just felt there was a terrible need to help save the animals from this kind of tragic end, all those heads, legs, and tails of puppies, kittens, a terrier dog, and a calico cat brimming over the tops of the two trash cans.

I went home with a feeling of unshakable resolve that was so deep and so new that I could never speak about it to anyone. From that fateful day on, the road home was never the same. I knew that there was a new road beyond, and at the end of that long road, I too would have a veterinary degree after my name. There was nothing sentimental or romantic about this new life-road, because then as a child I could talk to the animals and they would talk to me. I understood them and I felt I could put myself in their place, and I could help them. I cared for many lost and stray dogs as a young boy, with my dear mother's help and encouragement, and my father's when he was on leave from military service during the difficult war years when food was rationed and money scarce.

I was fourteen and that war was over when one of the local veterinarians, Donald Routledge, came to our home to treat Raq, our Welsh terrier mix who had cut his paw badly. He was a stocky Scotsman, a World War II veteran, and his tweed jacket and corduroys smelled of cow barns, pipe smoke and sheep sheds. After he had attended to my dog, my mother offered him tea. But somehow he was soon settling down to a second shot of scotch, lighting his pipe and telling me that since my mother says I want to be a veterinary surgeon some day, perhaps I would like to accompany him on his rounds on the weekends. And that I did for several years until I entered veterinary college.

I learned much on my Sunday rounds with Mr. Routledge during my teenage years. By the time I graduated from high school and gained admission to the Royal Veterinary College, London, I had considerable practical experience that was invaluable, especially in my pre-clinical years that seemed so far removed from helping sick and injured animals. It was this knowledge that too many of my teachers lacked, and the sterile environment of the college classrooms combined to make the five years of study an ordeal to forget. Fortunately, there were some illuminating childhood experiences that helped me through these times, especially during the waking hours with Bruce, Rover, Gruff, and other owned and lost stray dogs who came into my life and were my companions, guides and teachers out in the fields and ponds around my neighborhood, and later, the Derbyshire dales and moors.

Before being admitted to the Royal Veterinary College, I was called in for an interview. Nervously seated before three elderly professors, I was anxious to display my knowledge and dedication. I correctly anticipated that they would ask me what the College's Latin motto "Veniente occurite morbo" meant, having had the foresight to ask my high school Latin teacher. "Meet death as it comes," I replied smugly, and they all laughed. "No, no my boy, meet disease as it comes, not death—disease."

Stunned, I retorted that I had, after all, asked my Latin teacher and that is what I had been told. I added that I found their translation no improvement since it would be better, would it not, to prevent disease rather then "meet it as it comes."

They looked at each other and then at me in silence, and then the one who seemed to be in charge, whom I later learned was Professor Burrows, head of pathology, looked over his half-moon, steel-rimmed glasses and said "Thank you, Mr.—er—Fox, that will be all. You will be notified in due course."

I was soon notified, after a seemingly interminable wait, that I had been accepted, and endured five years of mainly memorizing from books and lectures and regurgitating the contents at intervals when I was given oral and written exams. At Finals, pre-graduation examinations, which many class-mates failed, I faced the very same Prof. Burrows. He asked me to define pathology, and word quickly spread that he was floored by my answer that, "it is the hand-maid of medicine and the servant of surgery." It was not the answer he expected.

What kept me going through those five interminable years was "seeing practice," going on farm visits and house calls with veterinarians in different parts of the country and helping in the hospital during surgery and clinic hours. The books and the lectures and the science had so little to do with the real world, with human-animal relations. Or with animals' behavior and how good understanding, empathy, and compassion made the difference between health and disease. After graduating from the Royal Veterinary College, London, in 1962, I spent several years studying and teaching animal behavior and development that eventually led to a tenured position at Washington University in St. Louis. My wolf research in particular opened me to the plight of this highly evolved species, and with growing concern over the treatment of captive wild animals, the mistreatment of 'factory' farmed animals and of those used in biomedical research, I realized the need for an integrative science of Animal Welfare. This would be an interdisciplinary field of animal behavior/ethology, ethics, and veterinary medicine. In order to become more of an advocate for animal rights, I left academia in 1976 to work full-time in the animal protection movement.

Now for over 30 years I have been writing the syndicated newspaper column "Animal Doctor." This column has taught me much about peoples' attitudes toward animals, the emotional and behavioral problems animals may develop, and the similarities of many of their health problems with those afflicting the human population. In addition, my investigations of how farmed, laboratory, zoo and circus animals in particular are treated have helped me gain further insights into human nature and the nature of disease.

With this background sketch of my professional experience, I offer the following testimony and testament for the animals and the environment/natural world we share with them.

CHAPTER 2
A Veterinarian's Personal Manifesto

I have worked on many fronts over the past several decades addressing some of the harmful consequences of unbridled anthropocentrism. This is a condition where self-interest precludes consideration and concern for the interests of others, human and nonhuman. At a talk by H.H. the Dalai Lama, he advised that if we must be selfish, then at least let us be altruistic. Altruism is the highest form of human selfishness. It is an enlightened selfishness when that altruism encompasses all living beings, even those whom we may fear and which could cause harm, and also the natural environment. This is the antidote to pathological anthropocentrism of culture and civilization, as it is the remedy for our collective narcissism, greed, indifference, hatred, and a host of other harmful consequences of human ignorance and fear.

All things causing disease, disharmony, imbalance, (what the Hopis call koyaanasqatsi) are connected, the co-factors of disease being now primarily anthropogenic. Americans, for example, actually underwrite with their tax dollars the production costs and market support prices of commodity crops and animal products that are part of the industrialized food system that costs them their health and their lives. This system is a major co-factor of climate change, and cases irreparable environmental destruction and pollution, as well as animal cruelty and suffering, and species and habitat extinction.

A medicine based on the humility and respectfulness of enlightened selfishness first seeks to understand the nature of disease and the often reflective, concurrent disease in nature before deciding how best to heal and prevent dis-ease. When we harm the environment, we harm ourselves, and when we abuse animals we do no less to our own humanity. Earth-care, animal care, and human care are coins of the same ethical currency as are earth-health, animal health and human health. All good farmers, physicians and veterinarians embrace these principles, but none could stop the juggernaut of industrial agriculture and cruel factory farms which organized veterinary medicine saw as progress.

It is no coincidence that we now face our own nemesis, or nature's retribution, because of our adversarial attitude toward life. This has lead to the evolution of antibiotic-resistant strains of bacteria, insecticide-resistant insects, and herbicide-resistant 'superweeds', notably to Monsanto's globally marketed herbicide called Roundup.

Civilization is a biological, evolutionary process, and we atom-splitting, gene splicing apes are learning that it is founded and sustained not by power, control, law and order, but by mutual respect, cooperation, humility and fairness, qualities and principles of being civil that we extend to all living beings because we feel for them and recognize them as members of the same life-community. Animals are as much Earth-citizens as are we. So, by extension, regardless of any claim we may have over them, they all have a life of their own. Our duty to care for animals under our dominion is to insure that their basic needs are met, just as we seek the same for ourselves, and which are the basic rights of all members of the life community.

There are many who feel no kinship with other living beings and who are uncivil toward them, showing varying degrees of biopathic behavior, much like the sociopath towards other humans. Regrettably, biopathic behavior has become the cultural norm for industrial civilizations and imperialistic corporations for which the natural world is simply a material resource, animals are mere commodities, a means to an end rather than being ends in themselves. Harvard biologist E. O. Wilson's appeal for biophilia and 'conciliation' with Nature notwithstanding, those core values and perceptions underlying biopathic activities and policies call for the application of bioethics to evaluate and guide all human institutions, both religious and secular. Bioethical principles such as equalitarianism, respect for all life, and ahimsa (avoiding harm) can make our altruism enlightened and our economies sustainable. But they are just as easily ignored behind a corporate façade of biophilia. Animal suffering in the biomedical research and product development laboratories is justified on the false grounds of human necessity, just like the cruel animal factories are rationalized as being necessary to meet market demand for 'affordable' food. The ethical vacuum of such animal use and abuse is made possible by the moral inversion of anthropocentrism, which gives sanction to such biopathic mistreatment of other sentient beings. We are told that is all for our own good, or for the good of society, the economy, or medical progress.

Those who speak the universal language of compassion act from the heart of an empathy-based ethics and a justice-based morality infused with understanding and loving concern. Ascent toward a more enlightened humanitarianism out of the spreading mire of barbarism in every form, secular and otherwise, with its moral inversions, nihilism, denial and corruption of spirit and purpose, requires more than choice and chance, science and faith. It calls for courage, conviction, absolute commitment and dedication to those bioethical principles that frame our humanity and which, like reverence, compassion, loyalty, and honesty, are absolutes, or they are not at all.

When our power of will is aligned with the Golden rule, it is greater than the will to power and rule of gold. Then the evolution of a wiser and more humane species worthy of the name Homo sapiens may proceed, and avert the extinction-possibilities of another millennium of unbridled anthropocentrism.

The above concerns and assertions will be revisited in subsequent chapters and addenda and examined more thoroughly with supportive documentation where appropriate and available. The care and welfare of companion animals will be examined especially from the perspectives of breeding practices which tend to propagate heritable diseases; the harmful consequences of them being over-vaccinated and fed manufactured pet foods, many of which are linked to serious health problems, and the role of the veterinarian where conflicts of interest are considered, and considerable. Solutions will offered and the groundwork laid for a more integrative, holistic approach to pet health care and disease prevention.

Bound by even greater economic and political forces, the health and welfare of animals raised for food are even more challenging issues for concerned veterinarians and consumers alike. How they are raised, and our food produced by the 'agribusiness' food industry, including the wholesale use of agrichemicals on crops and their genetic engineering, along with the cloning of genetically modified farmed animals, are complex subjects that will be discussed in depth. Industrial and other nonsustainable farming practices that have profound environmental impacts and affect wildlife and biodiversity will also be addressed.

Solutions to these issues and concerns, based on sound science, sustainable economics and bioethics, will be outlined as an enlightened approach to human health and well-being, contingent upon healing of our relationships with animals and the natural world.

CHAPTER 3
How Animals Suffer Around the World

I am often asked what are the worst kinds of animal suffering in the world today? With over 50 years experience as a veterinarian and animal care advocate working in the US and in poor third world countries, I offer the following review. This will, I hope, encourage international efforts focusing on improving the human condition to also address animal concerns because Human Wellbeing means HealthCare + PeopleCare + AnimalCare + EarthCare. In other words, a healthy population of domestic animals improves public health and livestock-based economics, and a healthy population of domestic animals means fewer diseases being spread to wildlife, an aspect of conservation that is too often neglected.

This review will also help encourage donors, from both private and corporate and government sectors, to give more support to animal care and protection worldwide, and dispel the erroneous view that people must come first and that human well-being has no connection with animal care and protection.

Animal suffering is a worldwide problem. Most of their suffering is associated with human poverty – insufficient resources to care for animals – as well as human ignorance, indifference, need and greed. Progress in animal welfare and protection, and ultimately liberation of animals from cruel domination and exploitation, entails greater public recognition of the

As we rank animal suffering in terms of severity, we must consider the duration of suffering, especially the deprivation of basic physical and psychological needs, chronic diseases, malnutrition and cruel methods of human domination and control.

In the wild, animal suffering is minimized by predation where carnivores kill and consume sick, aged and injured animals and help regulate herbivore numbers and prevent habitat destruction from overpopulation/overgrazing. But wildlife suffer from a host of human influences, from habitat encroachment and destruction, and fall victim to trapping, hunting, poisoning, and diseases spread from infected domestic animals who compete with wild herbivores for food and with wild carnivores for prey.

While the extinction process is being accelerated for wildlife by these and other anthropogenic factors, including global warming, agrichemical poisons and industrial pollution, the plight of domestic animals is no less pervasive around the world; and their suffering is more severe because their lives are not mercifully and swiftly ended by natural predators. Instead, their existence and suffering continue because of various human influences, be it the garbage that keep third world dogs and much livestock alive; and the antibiotics and vaccines that keep factory farmed livestock alive to grow quickly for slaughter.

First, I would rank third world street dogs, in terms of the sheer duration and degree of agony that the animals suffer, and in view of the numbers of animals so suffering. Millions are slowly eaten alive by mange, maggots, and internal parasites, and endure only so long as they can find enough food so that they do not die from starvation first, or before rabies or distemper puts an end to their lives.

Some of these common diseases that are easily prevented are frequently transmitted to humans, especially children. Consequently, dogs who are sick are often shunned, stoned, and clubbed. In order to control such zoonotic diseases, both sick and healthy free-roaming dogs are often poisoned by local authorities with strychnine, or are caught and killed with an injection of Epsom salts, or are electrocuted, drowned, or killed with engine exhaust fumes. Periodic dog roundups and the killing of dogs, many of whom are owned and valued by the community, cause much anguish especially to children who witness the mass dog massacres. In the absence of spay, neuter and vaccination programs, these mass dog killings must be repeated at regular intervals as the dog population increases.

Second, I would rank especially the plight of the beasts of burden in the third world – the goaded and overburdened donkeys and bullocks (oxen), ponies and water buffalo. Veterinary services are either too costly, or not available when needed for most of these poor creatures, who, if too ill or crippled and malnourished to work anymore, are simply abandoned to fend for themselves.

Third, I would rank all the billions of livestock in the third world who suffer seasonal starvation, die from thirst, and from the many diseases that they too often spread to wildlife with devastating consequences. The suffering of cattle, buffalo, goats and sheep is aggravated by chronic overgrazing and lack of adequate feed and veterinary care in most developing countries, and especially for the "sacred" cows of India where the religious taboo against slaughter means slow death from malnutrition and disease for millions of discarded, nonproductive cattle.

Fourth, I would place the billions of intensively raised, commercially exploited creatures raised on factory farms for their eggs, flesh, fur, and for their off- springs' own milk, and for various medical products (like pregnant mare urine and bile from bears in China). In this fourth rank are all creatures who spend their lives incarcerated in small zoo and circus enclosures and cages, or spend a life in chains like the working and temple elephants, who have been beaten until their spirits are broken into obedience. Also in fourth place I put the millions of animals—mice, monkeys, cats and dogs—who live their entire lives in small cages and are bred and used in often unnecessary and painful medical and military research experiments, and in product safety tests.

Fifth, the short-term suffering of various wild animals that humans kill, notably the whales who are harpooned; those species that are trapped for their fur, shot by nonsubsistence "sports" and trophy hunters, and predators like panthers and coyotes who are poisoned or killed by other cruel means by government and private agents, fill the fifth category of animal suffering in the global holocaust of the animals.

Sixth, the confined, often overfed "pets" of the affluent sectors of first and third world countries, from guinea pigs and parrots to poodles and parakeets, who are too often deprived of any contact with their own kind, are being forced to live in small cages for most, if not all, of their lives.

There are many other human uses and abuses of animals, from horse and greyhound racing and bull fighting and dog and cock fighting, to animal circuses and "canned" trophy hunting, that can be added to the above holocaust list and categorization in terms of severity of suffering. The justification/rationalization of human need, be it economic, scientific-medical, or emotional and social/traditional, for the continued exploitation and suffering of animals, be it long- or short-term, must be examined from a bioethical perspective. From this perspective, we ask is it necessary, is it avoidable, and are there alternatives to satisfy our needs and wants that will eliminate or minimize the suffering of animals?

The fatalistic acceptance of animal suffering in poor countries is linked with the hopelessness of people, often oppressed, living in abject poverty. The politics of animal welfare and liberation, and wildlife conservation, are closely tied to the human condition. Human overpopulation and poverty are only part of the problem. Corruption and misappropriation of funds and other resources to help people and animals are major factors that many governments and nongovernment organizations continue to deny or discount, and blame all on human poverty and overpopulation, which is used as a scapegoat.

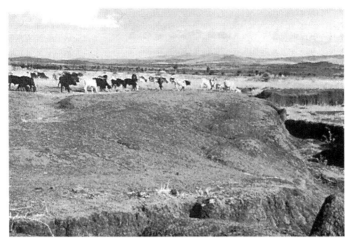

Figure 3-1. Erosion from Overgrazing Livestock in Tanzania
(M.W. Fox)

Our perception of animals determines how we treat them and whether they suffer under our dominion or not. Behind our perception and treatment of animals lie our needs, wants, values, and cultural and religious traditions. Until these are addressed, and our perception changed so that there is empathy, respect and communion, the holocaust of the animal kingdom will continue: And those qualities or virtues that make us human – humility, compassion and selfless benevolence – will continue to be crushed by the arrogance, ignorance and selfishness of our species.

CHAPTER 4
Harm and Be Harmed

It seems that we do not learn that when we harm the Earth and other living beings, we will as a consequence harm ourselves. This may be a universal principle, a kind of natural law, which like the Golden Rule, is enlightened self-interest to obey. It does seem like Nature's retribution when people drown or are buried under mudslides after they have deforested the hillsides around their villages and there are no trees to hold the rains and the soil.

Bacteria and insects strike back with force after they become resistant to all the antibiotics and pesticides we have used so indiscriminately and without any concern or respect for these "lower" life forms.

Creating new, alien life forms by putting the genes of one species, like a fish, a bacterium or a human, into another species, like a tomato, a corn plant or a pig, is to harm the natural order. It is a violation of the sanctity of life, of species' biological integrity, ecological fitness and evolutionary status. The consequential harms to humanity of this new technology are yet to come. The first intimations — allergies to new foods, genetic pollution (where the pollen of genetically engineered crops contaminate natural crops) and the destruction of beneficial insects by crops engineered to produce their own pesticides do not bode well. They affirm the dictum "harm and be harmed."

The retribution of "higher" life forms like dogs, pigs, chickens and monkeys against those who harm them is less immediately obvious. Highly infectious and often fatal diseases, like Ebola, Hanta, and the plague, are often associated with human activities that disrupt the habitats, populations and movements of wildlife, either directly through deforestation and killing natural predators, or indirectly via global warming, for example.

Twenty years ago I was lambasted as a jeremiad for predicting the harmful consequences of intensive livestock production factories and feedlots: these included untold animal suffering and disease, environmental pollution, the demise of rural communities and new food-borne plagues. But my predictions were based on science and reason, not on some prophetic doom and gloom vision behind which was some hidden vegetarian or other nefarious agenda as my detractors claimed.

To be prophetic in the face of denial and rationalization by supporters of the livestock industry, including many of my peers in the veterinary profession, who claimed farm animals don't suffer in confinement and that factory farming is the only way to feed the hungry world, is to experience alienation and outrage, and then pity and despair. Was it not obvious when factory farming began in the 1950s that confined, overcrowded and stressed pigs, chickens and cattle would suffer from immune system impairment, develop new diseases and become incubators for potentially harmful diseases (zoonoses) affecting humans and wildlife? Virulent strains of Salmonella and E. coli sicken millions of people and kill thousands annually. These and other bacterial and viral diseases afflict wildlife. Penguins, for example, are being killed by poultry viruses from contaminated poultry offal dumped at sea off the coast of New Zealand.

Risk and Harm Determinations

Had the immediate harms of factory farming to the animals themselves not been denied and rationalized as the "price of progress" by agribusiness, these harmful consequences could have been averted. The evaluation of harmfulness entails the application of bioethics as well as good science and reason. Good science is holistic and interdisciplinary, and in the case of determining the harmfulness of intensive animal production, includes veterinary medicine, animal behavior and husbandry (not simply animal production science), economics, ecological science and social science.

Determining harmful causes and consequences is much more relevant and radically different from simplistic cost-benefit assessments. These are generally delinquent in considering the harms to others outside of the scope of concerns about investments and investors, public acceptance, profits, and competition. Actual and potential harms uncovered by risk assessments (as in the case of nuclear reactors, agricultural pesticides and genetically engineered crops) are of no ethical consequence when the anticipated profits outweigh the estimated risks. Lacking a science that can predict future events, we must err on the side of caution and common sense and not let greed and zeal and the arrogance of a little knowledge lead us to discount or deny the harmful and potentially harmful consequences of human activities and various products and processes. Such denial is a form of spiritual corruption that is so widespread today as to almost be the norm. We have been slow to learn that we cannot, with impunity, release unnatural amounts of natural substances (like carbon dioxide) or artificial and novel creations such as synthetic chemicals (like pesticides) and genetically modified organisms that are alien to the natural world into the environment and not expect the unnatural to have adverse effects on the natural. There are consequences far beyond our limited temporal, relational and molecular understanding of natural systems and processes. They lie outside of our capacity to do adequate risk assessments and to set up risk management protocols. Few, if any, experts expected fluorocarbons to destroy the ozone layer. Scientists in Europe, for example, have recently discovered that many prescription drugs that are eventually excreted in people's urine, are recycled back into the environment and can be found in drinking water. It is counter-intuitive, therefore, to wait until an unnatural substance causes harm and to deny the universal Precautionary Principle that some call the law of unforeseen consequences.

In any society where cruelty toward animals is condoned and ignored, there will also be more inhumanity toward humans and less respect for life in general than in a community where there is such respect for all life. How do we then create a community where there is reverential respect for life? Albert Schweitzer's ideal of reverence for all life has become a cliché. Empathy and compassion cannot be legislated when ethical principles and moral virtues are supplanted by the self-serving values of consumerism and global economism. Reverence for life has no place in the dominant materialistic culture of biological imperialism that is laying waste to the planet as it treats all of life as a commodity.

The ultimate nihilism of this worldview, the wastelands that it creates as well as the spiritual emptiness of the human condition, if not rationalized or denied, can serve to catalyze a transformation in human behavior and values. This transformation should be seen as enlightened self-interest, and that it is a survival imperative for all of us to realize that no life is merely a commodity, and that Nature is not simply a resource. When we believe so and act so, harming other lives and the natural environment, we inevitably harm ourselves. The ethico-spiritual leap to realizing that all of life is sacred and treating all living beings with reverential respect is too great for most to make. The first step is more utilitarian and is based on sound science and biological reality.

This step entails recognizing that every living being, from a tree and blade of grass to an earthworm and soil bacterium, are members of the life community. They all deserve equal and fair consideration because each contributes to health, maintenance, beauty, and evolution of the planet. Ecology is the scientific basis for the spirit of communitarianism and for the egalitarian bioethical principle of equalitarianism. It informs us that humans are different, not superior as a species over others; and since all species contribute to the life community (generally doing a better job than humans), they should be treated with equal consideration (eco-justice).

Heal and be Healed

The dictum "heal and be healed" is worth reflecting upon. When we enjoy a close emotional relationship with animals, their healing benefits to us and vice versa are evident and have been well documented. This indirectly supports the converse that when we are not close to animals and harm them, or are indifferent to their suffering, we harm our own humanity by impairing our ability to empathize. I also believe greater medical progress would be made if that state of mind that justifies performing painful experiments on animals was better informed about the "law of harmfulness."

We can also apply the same dictum "heal and be healed" to our relationships with wild nature and the environment. Restored ecosystems mean purer air and water and fewer floods and droughts. Restored soils ravaged by the chemicals and ecologically harmful consequences of industrial agriculture, healed by organic farming methods, mean healthier foods and safer drinking water.

Many bioethical principles and moral codes are derived from our long association with animals, plants and wild nature. In so-called primitive cultures anthropologists have often found a sophisticated understanding of ecology and a rich indigenous knowledge of plants and animals. Beneath seemingly irrational superstitious taboos was an appreciation of natural law and a nature-wisdom that sharply contrasted the ecological illiteracy and lack of ethical and moral concern for the natural world (and natural people) evident in western industrial society today; and in the colonialism of western empires of the past three centuries.

The indigenous knowledge systems of preindustrial civilizations included a practical as well as symbolic and totemic value and appreciation of local plants and animals. The arrival or departure of some migratory "indicator" species meant a change in the seasons for which the people would begin to prepare. Modern day ecologists refer to indicator species as those that, like the prairie falcon and tundra wolf, signal a diverse and healthy ecosystem that can support "apex" predators.

Animals also give us warning of danger. Like the proverbial canary down the mineshaft, the birth defects and extinction of amphibians around the world today has symbolic value to doomsayers and practical value to environmental toxicologists. But what of the intrinsic and extrinsic, biological value of these and other creatures now falling victim to myriad anthropogenic forces that are almost incomprehensible to the narrow, instrumental knowledge system of industrial civilization?

Industrialism and consumerism are based on extractive and distancing technologies and an economism that is driven by the values of efficiency and profits and the accumulation of wealth (capitalism). This contrasts the more appropriate technologies and self-sufficient economy of many indigenous peoples that enabled them to live less harmfully and more sustainably.

This was achieved by balancing the rate and quantity of extraction and consumption of natural resources with the regenerative capacities of the ecosystems they utilized and often enhanced through self-government, trial and error, and careful observation. Some pre-industrial societies learned how to enhance biodiversity and regenerative processes by developing highly sophisticated, ecologically sound methods of gathering, hunting, fishing, livestock grazing, crop production, food processing and storage/preservation. Their technologies may seem crude from the point of view of productivity, but in terms of maximizing the social good and minimizing ecological harm, they are highly sophisticated.

Ethical constraints may or may not correlate with the degree of technological sophistication. Primary constraints are identifiable in some pre-industrial cultures as virtues, like sharing, frugality, nonwastefulness, avoiding causing harm to other living things, and not despoiling the natural environment.

Harmlessness

Harmlessness is an ideal that is unattainable because in order to sustain our own lives as gently and mindfully as we can, we inevitably cause some harm to others. Life feeds upon life; life gives to life. But even though absolute harmlessness is an unattainable state, that is no reason to abandon it. Harmlessness is an ideal, a bioethical principle that can guide and inspire us to a more harmonious existence. The quest for power and control results in conflict and harm. The quest for understanding and harmlessness results in peace and harmony. So applying the bioethical principle of harmlessness equally to our political, industrial, agricultural and other secular institutions and spheres of commerce and interaction with each other and the natural world, is enlightened self interest. Otherwise we will continue to harm ourselves when we harm the Earth, as when we harm animals and other living beings.

When We Hurt for Other Beings

When we hurt for our own kind, for other animals, for trees, prairies and mountain lakes, what do we do? Why do some humans hurt while others feel nothing when they see wild Nature ravaged and animals suffering?

No one likes to feel hurt, and that is one reason why we try not to hurt others. By helping others who are suffering, we help alleviate some of the hurt we ourselves feel for them. We are also hurt when we see the beauty and integrity of Nature defiled. Some of those who feel this way about a forest being clear-cut or a hillside being blasted to extract coal, have a sense of being personally violated. In their deep heart's core, they feel harmed. Others react with moral outrage and a sense of injustice.

Not all empathic people are moved to action, however. Many just feel helpless, hopeless, depressed, until they find other kindred spirits for support, or are inspired to action by charismatic members of their community. Many people who care and would act are too afraid to do so. They face the specter of being ridiculed, of losing their jobs, and in some instances even their lives. Others stop caring because they have given up and surrendered in despair to man's inhumanity and callous disregard for Nature and all sentient life.

To surrender to the hurtful and harmful consequences of the evils that arise from the corruption of the human spirit will not make those evils go away. Evil indeed flourishes where good men do nothing. But evil is born where people do not hurt for others and have neither conscience nor concern when they harm others. Arising from abusive families and cultures, children who have been hurt and who have felt the hurt of others become adults who may avoid closeness for fear of being hurt, or find the only way to feel close or in control is to hurt others. A warning sign of this kind of pathology is when children and adolescents deliberately hurt animals and weaker peers. Rape and animal torture has less to do with sexuality and sadistic delight than with the perverted desire to dominate and hurt, born from suppressed and redirected rage and hurt.

That no good ends can come from evil means is an aphorism whose wisdom has been almost lost. To cause harm deliberately or out of ignorance, or to accept it as "unavoidable," like the suffering of animals in factory farms and in new product safety tests, is evil. Embracing the compassionate ethic of harmlessness is the antidote to the evils of human selfishness. Enlightened selfishness leads to altruism and to the realization that when we harm others, we harm ourselves.

The harms we cause as individuals may seem relatively insignificant within the scope of our own lives. But seen in the wider scope of our ever increasing numbers and exponential rise in consumer wants with industrialism, the collective harm of our personal lifestyles and consumer habits is apparent. The harmful consequences of our reproductive and consumptive impulses that are even protected constitutionally as inalienable rights and entitlements of every individual citizen, actually violate the rights and interests of future generations. They will suffer the harms of our overpopulation and over-consumption, inheriting an even more polluted planet depleted of natural resources and biodiversity, virtually devoid of any wild and unspoiled Nature. Compound these harms with the genetic and somatic damage to these future generations, and the psychic trauma of being born into a toxic environment and a dysfunctional society. But this apocalyptic prophesy need not come to pass since we all possess the power to change our ways and find in the ethic of harmlessness, a ray of hope for the generations to come.

Farmer and Physician Do No Harm

Most diseases are extremely complex. In only a few disease conditions like an acute attack of a very virulent strain of typhus, accidental pesticide poisoning, or inherited hemophilia, is there a single cause responsible for sickness and sometimes death.

Health is not simply the absence of disease. Disease, literally disease, is not a cause of human illness, something external that we "pick up." Rather disease is a symptom and consequence of imbalance, of some impairment in normal body function. An ecological or holistic approach to disease diagnosis, treatment, and prevention does not therefore focus on single-causes like a virus, or genetic anomaly, since most diseases are complex, a multiplicity of causal factors being involved in creating dis-ease. Lifestyles, eating habits, how our food is grown and processed, emotional and social distress and stress, all play a significant role in the genesis of most disease conditions as well as "bad" bugs, genes, and the medicines prescribed to treat some of the symptoms and which have iatrogenic (harmful) side effects. A holistic approach to human health entails the same reorientation in thinking, or "paradigm shift" in the medical profession that conventional farmers experience in their transition to humane, sustainable, organic agriculture practices.

Our thinking about disease is often as distorted as our ideas about death. Rev. Billy Graham says that "Death comes about because man has sinned." What happened then to death as a natural process? Doctors with a limited understanding of the nature of disease and health still fight life with death using chemical and biological weapons to kill or control potentially harmful organisms. Many harmless and beneficial organisms are harmed in the process, which can impair our immunity and stimulate the natural selection of more resistant and virulent life forms. The literal meaning of antibiotic is to be against life, which reflects the adversarial attitude toward illness which limits our ability to find better ways of disease prevention and treatment.

Doctors in England have recently encountered a mutated strain of enterococcus in patients' intestines that flourishes when the patients were given antibiotics. The bacteria had actually evolved a dependence on antibiotics to stimulate their metabolism and multiplication. According to Dr. Ian Eltringham, one of the physicians who made this discovery, "[The bacteria] could only survive if you gave it the antibiotic (vancomycin). The bug's poison became its food."

What most doctors do to our bodies in using steroids, antibiotics, and other drugs is like what most farmers do to their crops and livestock. Hippocrates cautioned doctors: physicians do no harm. Now I caution farmers to farm without harm: then fewer people will get sick.

Farmers destroy beneficial organisms in the living soil with agrochemicals just like doctors harm our beneficial intestinal microflora with antibiotics. Both doctors and farmers inadvertently encourage the proliferation of ever more harmful organisms and increase disease susceptibility in their patients, crops, and livestock. Poor soil quality as a result of monocrop farming and the use of agrochemicals leads to nutrient-deficient crops and a host of subsequent health problems in animal and human consumers.

So many of the complex diseases of contemporary civilization are not caused simply by "bad" bacteria, viruses and one's environment. They are in part the product and consequences of the monocultures of the food and drug industrial complex that is regulated, purportedly for the public good, by the FDA - the Food and Drug Administration of the United States government. Why one agency for food and drugs? Because both agriculture and medicine as currently practiced have a symbiotic relationship. People get sick from food lacking in essential nutrients, contaminated with chemical residues and fecal bacteria, and are then given various prescription drugs to correct these health problems. This linkage between the agribusiness and biomedical sectors of the expanding global monoculture of industrialism has been evident for several decades.

There are now more children being born with physical and neurological defects; more early cancers, immune system breakdowns, more allergies, chronic infections, attention deficit, affective and cognitive disorders, and lower IQs; and in adults, lower sperm counts, severe menstrual difficulties, and epidemic breast, ovarian, prostate, and colon cancer. In treating more and more of these diseases, doctors are finding many can be helped by a complete revision of the patients' and communities' dietary habits, and by finding more healthful food sources.

The adversarial approach to health and food security arises, I believe, from the deeply rooted fears in the human psyche of being helpless in the face of plagues, famines and pestilence, The aggressive profit motive is secondary, and no less damaging to the human body and the body-Earth. The adversarial and profit driven mind-set must be changed because it is neither reasonable nor scientifically sound. Nothing in Nature, or in our bodies, operates independently since biological systems are interconnected in many ways. Thus any new element, be it an antibiotic, a synthetic fertilizer, or a genetically engineered organism that is released will have unforeseeable and possibly harmful consequences. The cavalier attitude toward new agrobiotechnology products like synthetic bovine growth hormone (rBGH) and herbicide, virus and insect resistant crops is of concern to many. Genetically engineered bacteria like Klebsiella (used to make ethanol from corn husks) can proliferate in the soil and kill off other soil bacteria that help synthesize and transport nutrients to plants. Genetically engineered crops can transfer, via cross-pollination, their new traits to other related varieties, including weeds and purportedly organic crops. Those transgenic crops that produce insecticides, like Bt (Bacillus thurinogenesis), can lead to a more rapid selection of insecticide resistant insects.

We know nothing of the health consequences to nursing infants and fetuses of the insulin growth factor, which is elevated in the milk of rBGH-treated cows, or of genetically engineered soybeans now being put into infants' milk-formula. Nothing in Nature operates in a vacuum, and we should respect the law of unforeseen consequences and exercise more caution in what we put into the environment and indirectly into our bodies.

A vision of health, integrated eco-systems, and true prosperity are incompatible with the vision of industrial agriculture with its monocultures of genetically engineered commodities, animal factories and feedlots, and fragmented econosystems. This latter vision cannot be sustained when it harms the soil and all that grows and is sold to billions of humans to consume, from our daily bread, to the fancy "milk (and antibiotic) fed" veal that people continue to regard as bioethically acceptable food.

Bioethically acceptable food is all foods that have been produced in the least harmful ways to animals, to the environment and natural ecosystems in order to satisfy our basic nutritional needs. The cravings and status foods of many affluent cultures and of meat addicted, nutritionally ignorant people reflect a lack of bioethical constraint and sensibility.

Some bioethically acceptable foods are being more widely marketed under labels that say "natural" and "organic," but as yet consumers cannot rely on these labels. Few wholesalers and retailers can verify that the produce and food ingredients which they are distributing are indeed organic. Organic includes more than food safety and quality, and restricted use of crop and animal drugs and soil chemicals. It also means the adoption of humane and ecological principles and practices. That translates into active compassion toward all creatures and the adoption of alternatives to pesticides and factory farms. It also means working in harmony with nature. These are essential bioethical principles for both a sustainable agriculture and culture - as well as for the practice of safe and effective human and veterinary medicine.

As billions toil and fight for the next bowl of white rice or loaf of black bread, we see a quickening of our calamitous condition. Human fetuses before conception, via their primordial components inherent in father's sperm and mothers' eggs, have been damaged by our ignorance of natural systems, laws, causality, karma and consequences. Scientific hubris, bioethical illiteracy, and corporate greed have lead to the wholesale contamination of the biosphere with synthetic chemical and biochemical products and industrial byproduct pollutants. In accelerating the planet's metabolic rate by burning fossil fuels, we are disrupting the atmosphere, regional climates, biological seasons, and rhythms, all of which harms all life and affects us adversely in body, mind, and spirit. The global economy and security of generations to come are also put in jeopardy. Our condition impels us to understand the true nature of reality, refine the sciences of survival and security, and practice the acts of benevolence, compassion, and reverence.

If instead we continue to harm any and all life in order to sustain the voracious and contrived appetites of industrialism, productionism and consumerism, the human species will die because as the Rev. Billy Graham said, "man has sinned." But that death as I see it is not the physical death that many fear. Rather it is our spiritual death. That spiritual death comes when we sacrifice all that is wild and natural in the process of creating an industrial monoculture through global environmental and biocultural rape and exploitation. In this twilight age between extinction and self-realization, the human species is left with one final choice, and that is between suicide and reverence for all life. We must make the right choices that are pro-life in a much broader sense of the word and in the knowledge that when we harm the cattle and other life forms, we ultimately harm ourselves. Some French gastronome, perhaps in a different spirit, once said "We are what we eat." Fortunately more doctors and parents are realizing this.

An auspicious beginning is the adoption of less harmful agricultural practices and treatments of crops, animals, and humans to prevent and treat a host of diseased conditions most of which we have brought upon ourselves.

Like the good holistic healer, the organic farmer treats the soil with the same reverential respect and nurturing compassionate understanding as the good veterinarian treats animals. But as the power of pesticides has replaced the wisdom of the farmer, so over-the-counter drugs, computers and gene-jockeys have replaced the eyes of a good stockman and the services of the livestock veterinarian. All these substitutions are costly inputs that have a multiplier effect that undermines the economic sustainability of farming enterprises that is being sacrificed as the off-farm sector of agribusiness reaps more profits from their products and services.

When industry and corporate America adopt the principles of bioethical responsibility, as exemplified by farmers who follow the ethics and scientific principles of humane, sustainable organic agriculture, and consumers and legislators support them exclusively and "eat with conscience," we will experience such healing that we will soon need no dietary supplements, like zinc and calcium, or vitamins C and E. We will have fewer cancers, heart attacks, babies with birth defects and children with neurological, cognitive and emotional disorders. We won't need pigs as organ donors, or legitimize the creation of transgenic animals that carry and suffer our genetic disorders to serve as profitable models for developing new drugs to treat the myriad diseases we have brought upon ourselves from cancer and chemo-sensitivity to immuno-suppression and auto-immune diseases. The replacement of animal-based foods with plant-based foods could result in an 80-90 percent reduction in cancer, according to Colin Campbell, Professor of Nutritional Biochemistry at Cornell University.

Culturally, we are so blindly disconnected from the metaphysical, the metaphorical and the spiritual, because we are cognitively and affectively immersed in the immediate, material, phenomenal world. We are as ensnared in matter as we are in our own materialism, egotism and our over-arching, all consuming anthropocentrism. When some problem arises, as in our own health or in the health and productivity of our crops and livestock, our perceptions are so limited and our motivation so often self-serving that we seek simple solutions — stronger antibiotics or genetically engineered, disease resistant seeds and stock — rather than correcting the underlying systemic causes. The expediency of simple solutions, often touted as miracles of scientific progress, serve the short-term, profit-oriented interests of the industrial system. The pathogenic status-quo is thus preserved for the benefit of a few at the expense of the many. This status-quo is crumbling, however, as people change their diets, rather than taking drugs to lower their cholesterol levels, and farmers turn to biological or natural methods of pest control.

Collectively, instead of seeking to understand complexity, we fear to embrace uncertainty and strive for control. We have no conception or resonant heart for concord and harmony with the life community. We slaughter dolphins, wolves, trees, and still even each other.

Our choice is to either extinguish this way of life or to extinguish all life that has no utility, no commercial value.

The less we cause animals to suffer, the less we will suffer. The less we harm Nature—the environment—the less we will harm ourselves, because, we and all life are connected ecologically, physically, psychologically and spiritually.

That most human diseases have a spiritual aspect has been long recognized by traditional healers. Conventional medicine does not address the spiritual, emotional, attitudinal, socio-ecological and economic dimensions of our dis-ease, or the many diseases of industrial civilization. It cannot be so long as it is ideologically, economically and politically part of the industrial system that it serves and services. It is a medicine that cannot prevent disease or heal, even the rich who can afford its ever more costly interventions, so long as it can justify its Professors of Progress and Experimental Surgery, removing the hearts of baboons and replacing them with the hearts of genetically-humanized pigs to see how long they might live before the monkey's immune systems predictably rejected these hearts.

What great step forward might such experiments on fellow creatures make for humanity? Is it not yet another backward step into the self-destructive morass of our once noble species turning into a global parasite, if not a plague on life more pernicious than AIDS? Such animal abuse and cruelty is endorsed by the Catholic Church, whose religious authority is embraced by the ruling bio-technocracy of the industrialized Western and Northern hemispheres to sanctify the commodization of animals and the wholesale, commercialized rape of what is left of the natural world.

The Eastern and Southern hemispheres are ensnared by the same pre-Copernican athropocentrism of industrial progress and economic growth that is to be attained regardless of the suffering of others, of the holocaust of the animal kingdom, the death of Nature, and the demise of indigenous peoples and their once sustainable economies.

We cannot put our faith and hopes in scientific discoveries that eventually prove how important the micro-organisms in the soil are for our crops to be healthy and our food nutritious: Or in new breakthroughs in agricultural and medical biotechnology. At best it will be too little, too late. More instrumental knowledge and technological advances will be to little avail if we do not shift the operational paradigm from anthropocentrism to a more reverential Earth or Creation-centered worldview.

We have yet to see that most of our diseases are not simply genetic or physical in nature, but also have a metaphorical aspect that has to do with our state of being and relationships with each other and with the Earth. The deterioration of our immune systems, for example, mirrors social and emotional stress and also the deterioration of the environment, of community values, and of the economy. That more holistically-oriented physicians are at last beginning to recognize these connections is a clear sign that a paradigm shift or change in our worldview is taking place and that the status-quo of conventional medicine, agriculture, the economy and other social institutions is no longer acceptable. As more medical scientists are becoming real healers, so more farmers are becoming real land-stewards. Their paradigm is based upon the following bioethical principles: compassion, humility, ahimsa (avoiding causing harm), reverential respect for all life; social justice; and eco-justice. These are the cornerstones of a healthy community and of a sustainable economy.

Advances in the science and bioethics of alternative human and veterinary medicine and agriculture that are based on this new paradigm hold much promise and should be supported by the corporate sector as well as by academia, the public and their governments worldwide.

The death of Nature will mean the death of humanity, since our humanity is derivative of the natural world, and has no primacy either in origin or significance. There is nothing miraculously different separating the existence of ants and earthworms from humans and tapeworms. All are different manifestations of being, of the life force. None is more significant, in itself, than any other in contributing to the diversity and dynamic harmony of the life process and community. It is from this perspective of a reverential respect for all life and for its community, that through communion, the time of healing will begin. This is a spiritual and ethical imperative, and a survival necessity for the human species in these times and at this stage in our evolution toward a wiser and more responsible, empathic and compassionate life form.

Some Radical Reconnections

Cancer is a complex and terrible disease that we are beginning to understand and to some extent more effectively diagnose, treat and prevent. We are learning to identify the anthropogenic (human-created) influences upon our immune systems of harmful chemicals, mineral deficient soils and nutrient deficient and imbalanced diets. We are also discovering the beneficial phytogenic influences of many different plant foods and herbal medicines and extracts on our immune systems, on our psyches and on cancer cells. These beneficial plant influences are weakened when the plants become unhealthy, nutrient deficient, and then vulnerable to pests and blights. Humans and other animals consuming such crops will also suffer the consequences of impoverished soils, weakened immune systems, and more epidemics, parasites, birth and growth defects, and anthropogenic diseases like cancer, and the new and complex autoimmune and immunodeficiency syndromes.

We are discovering that when wee supplement our diets with antioxidants like Vitamin C, the Bioflavonoids, and Vitamin E, and increase our dietary intake of zinc, magnesium, and selenium, our immune systems function better. These and other supplements, coupled with medicinal herbal extracts like Echinacea, Astragalus root and Golden Seal are being ever more widely used by satisfied doctors, patients and self-healers. A change in diet to a well balanced, high fiber, organic vegan diet, seems to greatly facilitate the resolution and regression of some cancers and various other degenerative, anthropogenic diseases, and also contributes to the maintenance of health and vitality.

Blight-riddled wheat and parasite infested and disease prone livestock are "agricologenic" problems caused by various harmful agricultural practices. These plant and animal diseases are more easily prevented than treated. The prevention lies in a change in our worldview. This comes when we acknowledge all those health problems that are anthropogenic. When we harm the Earth we harm ourselves. Many of the preventives to these health problems are seen as a threat to various businesses — like everyone becoming vegan is certainly a threat to the meat and dairy industries. Some powerful vested interest groups, like the pharmaceutical, petrochemical, biotechnology and food industry complex, do not want to see farmers going organic and the consumer public becoming more responsible for their own health and aware of what makes them ill. They would like to see vitamin and mineral supplements available on prescription only, and have all the herbal, naturopathic and homeopathic remedies removed from the shelves.

But with a change in worldview, this multinational corporate complex, like others such as the mining, power and timber industries, can enrich their coffers and satisfy their investors, by developing and marketing ethical products and appropriate technologies. For products, technologies, and business practices to be ethically appropriate, there must be a new world view that provides a bioethical basis for the spirit of enterprise to do more good than harm.

The genetic engineers are discovering that genes do not function properly except in ultimate relationship with other genes, and with the environment, beginning at the enzymic, protoplasmic interface. It is at this interface we find the free radicals that damage DNA, and the place where certain vitamins and essential trace minerals neutralize free radicals and catalyze enzymatic processes, and cell and organ maintenance and repair.

These vitamins and trace minerals are essentially atomic, bioelectric particles of energy that are integral to the anabolic and catabolic processes of cells, organs, organisms and ecosystems. The natural flow and interplay of these energies, or "life-force," gives us our strength and vitality. Our own health and the resilience of our crops become dysfunctional and diseased when wee disrupt the flow of this force. We may also harm our minds, our basic faculties becoming so impaired that we fail to comprehend the anthropogenic nature of disease and ecological disintegration: Like our ancestors who cleared the mountain forests to make iron and bricks, war and cities, and died in floods, famines, droughts, and suffocated from the poisonous gases and ashes from volcanoes and factory chimney stacks.

Dioxins, from some of these modern incinerator stacks, now put consumers of French Camembert and other cheese at risk and also those who eat deep-sea fish and range-raised beef and lamb. These consumers put their offspring at risk too, since nursing infants and developing fetuses are especially sensitive to dioxins, pesticides and heavy metal contaminants, and other chemical energy particles that disrupt and block the flow of the Life-force in our cellular, neuro-hormonal, metabolic and reproductive systems.

So as we say to the physician, first heal thyself and do no harm, so those who farm should first feed themselves, and do no harm. The Earth is our flesh and from stones we can make bread. When we start to heal the Earth, only then will we begin to heal ourselves. As the Zen poet saw, "Rocks are peopling rocks."

Radical Disconnections

I see cancer as one symptom of a widespread phenomenon that I call radical disconnectedness. When certain cells become disconnected from the gene-mediated regulation of cell growth and differentiation, they either die or become neoplastic.

Some of the anthropogenic factors contributing to poor crop, livestock and consumer health fall in this category of radical disconnectedness. The solution therefore lies in making radical reconnections, which is what organic agriculture and holistic human and veterinary medicine are all about. For instance, we radically disconnect crops from the good Earth by not replenishing the soil with rock minerals and manures that make organic humus. Conventional agrichemical-based farming kills the life in the soil, notably plant root mycorrhizas and soil-making earthworms and other invertebrate creatures and micro-organisms. Potentially harmful organisms become like cancer cells, proliferating in a sick ecosystem like neoplastic cells in a sick body. Similarly, antibiotics in livestock feed can lead to the proliferation of harmful, resistant strains as beneficial species are wiped out. These radical disconnections of crops from what was once good earth have a domino effect on the health of those humans and other animals who consume them.

Another serious radical disconnection is exemplified by intensive confinement methods of livestock production. Animals are no longer an integral part of land and resource management and of ecologically integrated crop, livestock and fodder production - often being located many miles from where their feed is grown. The solution is organic farming that utilizes livestock for its primary ecological role in sustainable agriculture. Yet another radical disconnection that community supported agriculture is rectifying is the disconnect between producer and consumer.

A no less egregious, if not heinous radical disconnection is in our depriving plants (hydroponic) and animals (factory contained livestock) from the sun, whose full spectrum radiation most plants and diurnal animals depend upon. Then I too feel for these poor animals, so radically disconnected from the Earth and made so helpless, with no control over their environment. They are deprived of the opportunity to forage what beneficial herbs in their wisdom they may desire, and good dirt to eat too, as they often must. Where now are the good earth and the herbs, except on the heirloom family farm of generations ago, and on some organic farms? Surely nowhere else in the biological deserts and industrial wastelands that agribusiness is making around the world.

Of course, one of the most radical disconnections in the "civilized" world is between consumers and the soil, the organic wastes of the former being diverted from fertilizing the latter by the flush toilet. The end result is pollution of coastal waters or contamination of farm land by municipal sewage often toxic with heavy metals and other chemicals.

We also have examples of radically wrong connections, like feeding some 40 billion pounds of farm animal remains back to farm animals, turning cows into cannibals, and putting an entire population of British beef eaters at risk from mad cow disease.

It is through bioethics that we may begin to restore our animal and environmental connections which ultimately benefit human health and well-being. The next chapter explores how ethics, based on sound biological science and empathy, expands the scope of our moral concern for the benefit of all.

CHAPTER 5
The One Medicine, Veterinary Bioethics & Planetary Health

PART 1

The science and practice of human and veterinary medicine are being re-defined by such global issues as global warming/ climate change; rising world hunger and poverty; the many complexities of zoonotic and other infectious and contagious diseases; species and habitat extinction; and food-safety and security in times of terrorism and war. The linkage of such issues and concerns are bringing human and veterinary medicine together in new ways that are being referred to in the professional literature as 'the one medicine'.

Resolving The Veterinary Dilemma: People Or Animals First?

A major bioethical dilemma facing the veterinary profession today is how to respond to a growing public demand for improved treatment of animals in society, especially those who are exploited for commercial purposes, from biomedical research to food production, and the mass production of pure breed dogs in puppy mills, as well as the mistreatment of wild animals in circuses and many zoos. There would be no dilemma if economic concerns took second place to animal welfare, and if sectors of the veterinary profession were not aligned with those vested interests in maintaining and expanding an increasingly global market economy based on animal exploitation. Fundamentally it is the consequence of anthropocentrism that leads us to regard and treat other animals as inferior. This perception is now becoming more zoo-centric, where animals are appreciated and respected in their own right and light. This means that making interpretations of their emotional and motivational states that seem anthropomorphic are no longer taboo, (Balcome 2006, Bekoff 2007).

Human ignorance, customs and conventional attitudes toward animals notwithstanding, the domestication and commoditization of once wild animals, who have not all lost their entire ethos or original natures, and are therefore not yet adapted to the kinds of environments and ways of treatment to which we subject them for pecuniary ends, is a long neglected bioethical issue: And a conundrum. How can we claim, as a society, to care for animals, when economic interests take precedence over animals' welfare and overall well being?

That our domesticated animals' ancestors were taken originally from the wild for the purpose of domestication is a fact that we must all consider when addressing animals' adaptive capacities. The welfare and wellbeing of domesticated animals are compromised as when the highly productive varieties of pigs, cattle, poultry, fish, and other species, all genetically altered to varying degrees, are forced to live in totally unnatural, stressful conditions, (Webster 2005). These can range from almost total physical restriction and environmental impoverishment, as is the case for breeding sows and most veal calves, (ditto too many wild animals in zoo and circus cages), or extreme overcrowding, as is the case with battery caged laying hens, farmed salmon in floating net-cages, and piglets in confinement stalls and pens, (Fox 1997).

The narrow view of human health as being the absence of disease has been long redundant with the World Health Organization. Likewise the narrow view that the absence of disease in animals, especially those that are raised for human consumption, is a cardinal indicator of health and overall wellbeing is untenable. The truth is that their health depends so much on the use of vaccines and an armament of drugs that can have serious adverse environmental, public/consumer health, and long term economic consequences, and this situation is no longer tenable. Such treatments are not based on sound science, but on the animal productivity paradigm of agribusiness' economism that is devoid of any bioethical framework. A blatant example of economic concerns trumping animal welfare concerns is in the transportation of pigs to slaughter, where the economies of transportation justify extreme overcrowding that can result in some economic losses when some pigs succumb to the stress and their carcasses become unfit for human consumption (so called 'slimy cutters'). Likewise the economies of scale justify large dairy herds, huge hog and poultry factories, and massive beef and dairy feedlots. But the costs in animal welfare and health, as well as the environmental and increasing public health costs, (Hu and Willett 1998, Campbell 2005) have been too long discounted.

To reason that antibiotic and other drug and vaccination maintained confinement sheds containing thousands of pigs or poultry are acceptable from an animal welfare perspective because the animals are productive (the pigs and poultry grow quickly and the hens lay many eggs), and disease incidence is low, is patently absurd. Animal health determination includes psychological as well as physical well being, not simply the absence of disease. Animal health and animal welfare are co-dependent. One cannot be taken away without affecting the other. Likewise, animal welfare standards must consider not only animals' physical needs and requirements, but also the related psychological/ emotional/, behavioral, social and environmental needs (McMillan 2005, Webster 2005).

The labyrinth of animal cruelty and suffering, and ways we follow in the destruction of the natural world, differ from culture to culture and age to age, as likewise the recognition of human rights, social justice, and the ethical imperatives of animal and environmental protection. The deeper into this psycho-historical labyrinth of inhumanity toward animals we journey, the more we find it leading to no less indifference and cruelties toward our own kind —not the individual psychopathic aberrations of the animal mutilators and serial killers, —but in the collective acceptance and institutionalized execution of no less cruel and debasing, if not as immoral abuses like human slavery, political imprisonment and torture; animal experimentation, factory farming for fur, and flesh, milk and eggs; and cultural traditions like the bull fight, bear-baiting, whaling, and turning captive elephants, tigers, and other wild and endangered species, in to circus performers.

The concept of the 'one medicine' that is emerging as veterinary and human medical fields converge and collaborate with particular emphasis on environmental, indeed planetary health, will only succeed if equal consideration is given to the treatment and alleviation of the symptoms of dis-ease as it is to the prevention of harm and suffering to all sentient beings that contribute to the functional integrity of the Earth's ecology, as well as to the life and beauty of the Earth. We have been slow to learn that when we harm the bacteria in our digestive systems and in the soil, we harm ourselves and our crops.

Such prevention goes way beyond better vaccinations and diagnostics, to examining our values and relationships, as in how the land and farmed animals are treated, along with the crops and foods we and they consume. Preventive medicine must also examine, like the shamans and healers of past civilizations, the icons and totems associated with the more destructive and harmful dimensions of the cultural ethos and human psyche. Physician Albert Schweitzer's (1965) remedy that he prescribed for many of the world's ills was based on such a holistic view of human well-being, namely, reverence for all life. But if reverence is conditional or partial rather than absolute and all embracing, it can be no more than feel-good paternalism, and a sentimentalist illusion.

Global Issues and Bioethical Perspectives

Part of the now global, systemic pathology of increasingly dysfunctional terrestrial and aquatic ecosystems parallels the condition of local and national resources and economies (Goodland 1997, Imhoff and Baumgartner 2006). The catalysts and vectors of this pathology are multiple and synergistic (Diamond 2005). These include consumerism, industrialism, and human and domestic animal population expansion and concentration that combine to accelerate climate change, the loss of biodiversity, and the undermining of water and food quantity, quality, safety, and security (Korten 1995, Fox 1997).

The new 'life science' of genetic engineering biotechnology with its patented genetically modified (GM) seeds and transgenic and cloned livestock, seeking to capitalize on the world hunger and climate change crises, is more likely to worsen the situation. This is not only because GM crops are genetically unstable and so can spontaneously mutate to produce potentially toxic new protein compounds, (Wilson et al 2006, Domingo 2007): The application of this biotechnology is not consonant with ethics, and practices of more sustainable and humane farming systems (Fox 2004), many of which, in contrast to conventional agricultural practices, are economically more viable (Badgley et al 2007) , and produce more nutritious food with less harmful, and generally beneficial, environmental consequences, (Cooper et al 2007).

The contributions by some segments of the veterinary profession have a disastrous legacy. By direct and indirect association globally with the livestock industry and commodity crop producers, they are in part responsible for global warming/climate change, loss of biodiversity, and zoonotic diseases like swine and avian flu, E coli and Salmonella. Their combined roles in contaminating the food chain, oceans and rainwater with petrochemical fertilizers, pesticides, GMOs (genetically modified crops) and veterinary pharmaceuticals, are a matter of biological record—a legacy that will endure for generations, (Fox 2001, Steinfeld et al 2006). Many of these contaminants and pollutants are endocrine system disruptors and variously cause cancer/DNA cell damage, mutations, birth defects, infertility and harm the immune system.

Both conventional and complementary, holistic, alternative, and traditional (indigenous/native) agricultural, veterinary and comparative medical disciplines and traditions are now being utilized as valuable resources of knowledge and application to address some of the aforementioned concerns and issues. Other scientific disciplines and practices are being resourced also, such as environmental toxicology, immunology, reproductive, and molecular biology. Nutritional genomics (how nutrients influence gene expression and function) for companion and farmed animals, and applied ethology/animal behavior, essential to insure optimal well-being (health and welfare) for all captive wild, and confined domestic animals, especially those used in food production, biomedical research, and for other commercial purposes, are being integrated into human medical and veterinary practice and undergraduate education. As Einstein cautioned, (1954) 'The problems that exist in the world today cannot be solved by the level of thinking that created them'.

Evolutionary Adaptation or Extinction
From a holistic perspective it would be accurate to say that we and the world are one, being embedded in a co-creative matrix of mutually enhancing symbioses, (Margulis 1998) from the bacteria in our soils and digestive and dermal systems, to the sustainable economies of natural ecosystems and organic and biodynamic farming practices. Some scientists name this evolutionary period the Anthropocene epoch, since we discovered how to make fire, tools, and weapons to alter and exploit the world's habitats. This epoch is chronicled by the ages of pyrotechnology, mechanical, chemical, atomic and genetic engineering technologies and industries. The global crises that we face today can be seen optimistically as evolutionary challenges to our biology and psychology, shaping human nature for better or for worse, and for generations to come. When we harm the Earth we harm ourselves, and when we demean other sentient beings we demean our own humanity.

The lack of any unified sensibility in our regard for and treatment of animals and Nature, —the natural creation—means, in terms of child development, a schizophrenogenic environment for character formation and personality development. This may result in ethically inconsistent, morally compromised or inverted and emotionally conflicted perception and treatment of other sentient beings in adulthood. Totemic and iconic values and perceptions of animals and Nature range from the instrumental to the sentimental; from being objects of property, exploitation, and commerce, or subjects of affection, concern, and communion; and from treating others as ends in themselves, or to using them a means to one's own exclusive ends. Animals once feared or revered are now regarded variously as commodities, test-subjects, objects of scientific curiosity and potential economic or medical utility; as indicator and flagship species of ecological well-being, and as beloved companions and family members.

The 'golden mean' of mutually enhancing symbiotic and

commensal relationships is the iconic template for humane and responsible planetary trusteeship, and we have far to go ethically and legally before this state of being, where love and duty are one, is achieved. Such an achievement would herald the coming of what Thomas Berry (1988) calls the Ecozoic age, or, in the sense of this essay, the Ethicozoic age, where bioethics temper the anthropocentrism of the earlier industrial age of this Anthropozoic epoch.

Reverence for all life, in practice, means equalitarianism—giving all living beings equally fair consideration, especially in terms of the consequences of human values, appetites, actions, demands, and aspirations. It is synonymous with eco-justice. The new animal welfare legislation in the UK that mandates the 'duty of care' to animals under our dominion is a positive sign of the dawning of the Ethicozoic age.

Physician V.R. Potter (1971) first coined the term bioethics to link the biological sciences with ethics to demonstrate how bioethics can serve as a bridge linking ecology, environmental issues, medicine and public health. He was concerned that medical ethics was too narrowly focused. The same may be said of veterinary ethics (Rollin 2006) when there is no linkage with ecological and environmental science and consideration in the practice and teaching of veterinary medicine. Integrating the veterinary teaching curriculum with an empathy-based bioethical template (Fox, 1998 and 2006) would do much to meet the above challenges and issues related to the environment, animal health and welfare, and to the ultimate advancement of civilization.

Synopsis of Global Bioethics (From M.W. Fox, 2001)

1   Global bioethics calls us to give equally fair consideration to three spheres of moral concern:
    Human well-being (rights and interests)
    Nonhuman (animal and plant) well-being (rights and interests)
    Environmental well-being (biodiversity and ecosystemic integrity).
2   Global bioethics calls us to be accountable for our actions and appetites in relation to these three spheres; and to examine how well society, our politics, laws, economies (industry and commerce), religious, educational and other traditions and institutions, as well as our own personal lives, are in accord with the bioethical principles that unify these three spheres in the light and language of compassion, humility, and reverence for the sanctity of life.
3   Global bioethics calls us to actualize our natural, innate empathic sensitivity, moral sensibility and powers of reason, reflection, and

also self-control by embracing the precautionary principle.

4   Global bioethics calls us to consider the purpose and potentials of human existence, the significance of the virtues that make us human beings, and our duties and responsibilities for the Earth community, and for the integrity and future of Creation.

5   Global bioethics calls us to understand and respect the cultural ecology of moral pluralism and from this diversity of human beliefs, opinions, and desires, create a common ground of equalitarianism and respect for all life.

6   Global bioethics calls us to develop a unity of spirit for more effective and immediate crisis management, conflict resolution, and humane intervention where the compass of compassion directs reason and action toward world peace, justice, environmental and animal protection, conservation and restoration of biological and cultural diversity for the security and fulfillment of all sentient beings.

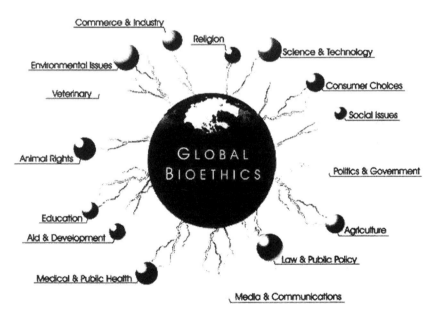

Figure 5-1. Global Bioethics (from *Bringing Life to Ethics,* M.W. Fox, 2001)

Global bioethics promotes and unifies an interdisciplinary, holistic approach to Health Care as the sum of Earth Care + People Care + Animal Care.

Table 5-1. Bioethics Seven Golden Rules

1. Compassion
2. Reverential Respect
3. Ahimsa (avoid harm/injury)
4. Social justice and trans-species democracy (equal and fair consideration)
5. Eco-justice/environmental ethics
6. Protect and enhance biocultural diversity
7. Sustainability

PART 2
Synopsis: Veterinary Bioethics in Practice— Feeling for Animals & Animal Feelings

Veterinary bioethics has a broader mandate than veterinary ethics that deals primarily with professional ethics and standards of practice. Veterinary bioethics addresses the ethos, telos and ecos of animals, namely animals' behavioral and emotional needs; their biological purpose, and, for domestic animals used for different purposes, their social, emotional and other uses or values; and their ecological, environmental roles, value and impact. It is commendable that the U.K.'s Farm Animal Welfare Council Chairman Professor Christopher Wathes has raised the animal welfare standards bar by invoking the concept of an animal deserving a life worth living, even if it is to be raised and killed for food. (See Viewpoint Lives worth living? Veterinary Record, April 10, 2010, p 468-469). This brings us closer to accepting that animals have interests, and therefore rights. Interestingly, author Wathes acknowledges the fact that subjective (affective) emotional states of animals can be recognized by veterinarians and experienced animal caretakers. This means that objective (impartial) determinations of animals' positive subjective states can be made (such as sociability, curiosity, playfulness, comfort/security, and contentment/relaxation), which in turn means that objective welfare standards can be applied to improve the quality of life of confined/captive animals.

Veterinary bioethics embraces the absolute moral principles of compassion and ahimsa, (avoiding harm), and is empathy-based, feeling for animals and recognition of animals' feelings being a prerequisite for optimal care, maximal animal well being, and welfare.

Many illnesses and behavioral problems in dogs, cats and also farmed, laboratory, circus and zoo animals can be prevented, and others cured by their caretakers/guardians adhering to five basic bioethical principles. These principles combine to make a simple formula to help insure animals' health and overall well being:

Right Understanding and Relationship + Right Breeding/ Genetics + Right Nutrition + Right Environment + Right Holistic Veterinary Care = Animal Health & Well-being.

It is every person's responsibility as an animal lover and/or care-provider to recognize the importance of these principles as basic animal rights for several reasons. These include the prevention and alleviation of much animal suffering; and reduced veterinary and other related costs associated with many animal health and behavioral problems, if not most, and even having to euthanize the animal or put her/him up for adoption.

These principles bring out the best qualities in people as caregivers by enhancing the human-nonhuman animal bond, and in the animals themselves under their care, in terms of quality of life and relational/emotional experience. They also provide an ethical compass of responsibility and compassion to advance the moral/character development of children, who, in learning by example how to respect and care for other animals, enhance their self-esteem and self-worth through loving service, and in the process refine their ability to empathize with other sentient beings.

As animals have served and benefited us for millennia and continue to do so in myriad ways, so we benefit the more we serve and help them as our wards, companions, healers, teachers, patients and friends— all of whom are related to us, but are more ancient, if not wiser than we. The bond that people have with the animals in their lives must become a boundless circle of compassion, expanding to encompass all living beings, domestic and wild, captive and free, if we are to justify keeping any animal as a domesticated companion beyond our selfish needs.

Veterinary bioethics calls on every veterinarian to apply the bioethical principle of compassionate care in their treatment of animal patients and in the advice given to client-owners and care-givers. This helps override the situational ethics of treating animals kept as commodities on factory farms where optimal care of animals on an individual basis is not normally provided for reasons of cost; and where a companion animal is not given optimal care because the owner is of limited financial means or does not feel that the animal is worth the expense of costly diagnostic and treatment procedures.

Rather than compromising their professional standards and integrity in such situations, veterinarians have a moral obligation to advocate compassionate care regardless of the context and situational ethics in which their services are required. This is because the bioethic of compassionate care is a fundamental human responsibility and every animal's basic right. Furthermore, compassionate care is vital to animals' health, welfare, and physical and psychological well being. It is therefore as essential a component of holistic, integrative, and preventive veterinary medicine as is caring for the land a vital aspect of sustainable agriculture.

Other professions and business enterprises are similarly being called to accountability and responsibility, just as all of us in our personal lives must find ways to cause less harm to the natural world and to animals domesticated and wild, in the process of satisfying our basic needs. To realize the long term benefits of applying bioethics in our decision-making and consumer-choices, to our own health, to the economy, and to the entire life community of this living earth, means living mindfully, and by the guiding principle of compassionate care.

No new laws, government oversight, or international conventions can equal the profound benefits that will come from the incorporation of the bioethics into the veterinary and medical teaching curricula, and into every level of society. Their relevance in rectifying conflicts of interest in the veterinary profession, yet to be more widely acknowledged, will be better appreciated after the following chapter, and subsequent discussion on what health care reforms and integrative (holistic) medicine really means for animal and human patients and their care-givers.

CHAPTER 6
Conflicts of Interest in the Veterinary Profession & the Origin of 'Man-made' Dog & Cat Diseases

Dogs are harmed more than cats by far too many veterinarians giving them unnecessary annual vaccinations. This can result in much suffering from several chronic health problems such as allergies, neurological and joint problems, autoimmune and endocrine diseases. Cats and dogs are prone to develop often fatal cancer (fibrosarcoma) at the site of vaccine injection.

Cats suffer more than dogs from poor nutrition because they are obligate carnivores requiring a meat-based diet. Too many veterinarians are profiting from selling dry cat foods high in cereals and soy that only too often lead to obesity, diabetes mellitus, urinary tract and inflammatory bowel disease and other chronic degenerative diseases. They then profit from treating these diseases and from prescribing expensive special diets that would not be needed if the cats were fed properly from the start.

But dogs are not without diet related problems that clear up once they are taken off highly processed manufactured foods that can be at the root of chronic skin and digestive problems, ear and anal gland infections, and a host of other maladies including depression and epilepsy.

Rather than addressing what their patients are eating, far too many veterinarians put them on cortisone/prednisone to stop self-mutilation from scratching and chewing. Then new health problems develop such as Cushing's disease in dogs and cystitis and diabetes in cats.

Veterinary dentistry has become a highly profitable field. An estimated seventy five percent of dogs in the US suffer from periodontal disease that is also a common affliction of cats. Many of these patients have such advanced dental disease that they may die on the operating table. Highly processed food ingredients that are micro-particulate, and especially the high cereal and gluten content of popular pet foods, play a major role in this virtual epidemic in the canine and feline population. Some veterinarians are advising pet owners to have their animals' teeth cleaned on an annual basis, and that typically means under general anesthesia that is far from risk-free.

Both dogs and cats suffer unnecessarily from adverse reactions to topical anti-flea and tick drugs that are widely promoted by many veterinarians, some being sold over-the counter (OTC) with no effective government oversight. Some OTC products are submitted voluntarily for review by the EPA, while all prescription products are assumed to be safer and better produced, when in fact not all are any better supervised or controlled. Topical prescription products are approved by the EPA, or in the case of systemic products, by the FDA. Better product labeling to help reduce adverse reactions in animals has been accomplished by the EPA after thousands of adverse reactions in dogs and cats were reviewed by this government agency.

Diseases of hereditary origin that result from inbreeding and selection for extreme traits in both dogs and cats add to this tragic burden of man-made diseases in companion animals today. The role of the veterinary profession in preventing such sickness and suffering in beloved dogs and cats should be central. But because of conflicts of interest, as between selling products for profit and putting the best interests of the animal patient before those of running a business, the veterinary profession bears similarities with the medical profession that have been called to question recently by the US Institute of Medicine. Such potential conflicts of interest go deep into the veterinary teaching curriculum where the influence of the multinational drug and pet food companies is evident at colleges around the world.

I sought to raise this issue of companion animal health and well-being and potential conflicts of interest in the following letter that I sent for publication in the professional journals of the British and American Veterinary Medical Associations, both of which I am a long-standing member.

Letter to the Editor,
Journal of the American Veterinary Medical Association,
Sent via e-mail May 26, 2009

Dear Sir,
EXAMINING CONFLICTS OF INTEREST IN THE VETERINARY PROFESSION
The relationships between the corporate sector, and in particular with drug companies, and private medical practitioners, hospitals, and medical schools, are being called to question by the Institute of Medicine in the US (1).

Is a similar examination called for in the veterinary sector where comparable corporate interests may be at play and affect the quality of care and services animal patients receive? It would seem that there has been a lack of due diligence over the role of diet, specifically, highly processed pet foods (2) in many contemporary health problems of companion animals. The same may be said about the routine application and so called 'preventive' treatments with anti-flea and tick topical products that only now are being fully evaluated by the Environmental Protection Agency (3). Was due diligence also lacking, in part because of inadequate information and understanding, with dog and cat vaccinations? Until recently the universal protocol of giving dogs and cats annual 'booster 'injections of multivalent live and genetically engineered vaccines met resistance when ever questioned.

Corporate sector partnering in academia even includes chairs and professorships named after the donating company at many veterinary colleges. What role such partnering may play in contributing to the grave consequences of poor diets, over-medication, and hyperimmunization in companion animals by deferring to vested interests and by claiming lack of scientific proof of harm from such practices, is an open question. Academia should not be exploited to garner public credibility, nor should the market place become the final arbiter of what is acceptable.

Examining possible conflicts of interest may be difficult, considering the partnership of the American Veterinary Medical Association with Fort Dodge and Merial pharmaceutical companies, and Hill's Pet Nutrition, who together have pledged $4.5 million in support of AVMA programs and services over the next four years (4). But this difficulty could become a confluence of interests once the health and well-being of companion animals are first and foremost on the agenda. The content of both the JAVMA, and its equivalent with the British Veterinary Association's (BVA) Veterinary Record, increasingly addresses issues concerning animal health and welfare, including nutrition and vaccinations.

In the UK, the government and the BVA have chosen to focus on the health and welfare problems of a genetic origin, primarily in pedigree dogs. Some critics believe that this is a massive displacement, since it is the genetic susceptibilities to dietary diseases and vaccinoses (adverse vaccination reactions) in specific breeds make them the canaries for the canine population at large (5). The appropriate use of vaccines, (6), various 'preventive' veterinary drugs, prescription diets, and the adequacies of manufactured cat and dog foods, also need to be considered if the mandate of the British government is to protect the health and welfare of companion and other animals, not just better regulate breeding practices. British dog breeders feel they are the scapegoats and are taking all the blame for the myriad and costly health problems in today's canine population. The same can be said for the major ailments in the feline population, where poor diets and adverse drug and vaccine reactions similarly take their toll according to Hill's former Director of Technical Affairs, veterinarian Dr. Elizabeth Hodgkins Esq.(7)

Of course there are confluences of interest that can benefit all and this would be forthcoming I believe when there is a more integrated approach to animal health and welfare. This could be developed from a bioethical basis (8) by veterinary teachers, researchers and practitioners, a Council for Veterinary Bioethics being one response to the call for an examination of possible conflicts of interest within the profession.

Letter References

(1) Sternbrook R. *Controlling Conflict of Interest—Proposals from the Institute of Medicine*. Published at www.nejm.org April 29th 2009 (10. 1056/NEJMp0810200).

(2) Fox M W, Elizabeth Hodgkins and Marion E. Smart. *Not Fit for a Dog: The Truth about Manufactured Dog and Cat Food*. Fresno, CA, Quill Driver Books, 2009.

(3) AVMA News. Topical flea and tick products come under EPA scrutiny. *J Am Vet Med Assoc* 2009; 234: 1228.

(4) AVMA News. AVMA enters into multimillion-dollar partnership with companies. *J Am Vet Med Assoc* 2008; 233: 219.

(5) Dodds WJ, Vaccination protocols for dogs predisposed to vaccine reactions. *J Am Animal Hosp Assoc* 2001; 38: 1-4.

(6) Schultz RD, Ford RB, Olsen J. and Scott F. Titer testing and vaccination: a new look at traditional practices. *Vet Med*, 2002, 97: 1-13 (insert).

(7) Hodgkins EM, *Your Cat: Simple New Secrets to a Longer, Stronger Life*. New York: Thomas Dunne Books, 2007.

(8) Fox MW. Veterinary bioethics, pp 673-678, in *Complementary and Alternative Medicine*, Schoen AM and Wynn SG. eds, St Louis, MO Mosby, 1998.

I did not even receive an acknowledgement from the British Veterinary Association, while the Interim Editor-in-Chief of the American Veterinary Medical Association's Journal of the American Veterinary Medical Association, that usually publishes my letters, sent me the following letter via regular mail, dated May 28, 2009:

> Dear Dr. Fox,
> Thank you for your recent letter to the editor. Although corporate influences on quality of care in the human and veterinary medical professions are important concerns, I am afraid that your letter attempts to address too many of these issues in too limited a space. Topics such as the effects of processed pet foods on the health of companion animals, annual vaccination of dogs and cats, corporate sponsorship of academic chairs and professorships, and the British Veterinary Association's focus on genetic diseases of dogs are so diverse and so complex that it is not possible to adequately discuss them all in a letter. Thus, I believe that readers will be confused as to the main point of your letter.
>
> For this reason, I have elected not to publish your letter. Please understand that this does not reflect a lack of concern about the topic, but simply my inability to understand what you are trying to convey to our readers.
> Sincerely, Kurt J. Matushek, DVM, MS, DACVS
> Interim Editor-in-Chief

What more can I say as a long-time advocate for all creatures great and small? I did not touch on the conflicts of interest in the veterinary sector that deals with farmed animals and which has pandered for decades to the interests of the livestock and poultry industries, placing the health and welfare of these animals in jeopardy. Organized veterinary medicine, that reaped great profits for the drug companies selling antibiotics, vaccines and a host of other drugs, never voiced concern over the proliferation of cruel factory farms, so call confinement animal feeding operations that now blight rural America, helped put family farms out of business and now pose significant environmental and public health risks. Ironically industrial animal agriculture has helped put the food animal veterinarian, who once served the nexus of productive family farms and ranches across the country, out of business.

It is ultimately enlightened self interest to use the moral compass of compassion and bioethics to avoid such conflicts of interest. There is no better example of this than in the food animal veterinary sector where animal welfare and health were sacrificed purely for profit under the erroneous banners of production efficiency, economies of scale and cheaper food for all. Now there is a shortage of new veterinary graduates entering this sector, and little wonder why, considering the working conditions and the kind of production-based medicine applied to stressed and over-crowded animals that should never be kept under such conditions in the first place. The corporate take-over of reason and sound science is one thing, but the apologists and instrumental rationalists of the rising biotechnocracy of transnational hegemony are a force that calls for a revolution indeed. And that begins with the spiritual anarchy of us all assuming greater responsibility for our own health and for that of our companion animals. A good beginning is in the market place and our kitchens with organically certified whole foods, and in our support of good doctors, animal and human, who practice integrative holistic medicine. To find a holistic veterinary medical practitioner in your area, a searchable list can be found at http://www.ahvma.org. Veterinarians wishing to learn more are encouraged to become members of the American Holistic Veterinary Medical Association at http://www.holisticvet.com

CHAPTER 7
What Real Health Care reform Entails: Animal & Environmental Protection, Food Safety, Security & Quality

The road to hell is paved with good intentions when vision is limited by ideology, and causes and consequences are ill considered. President Obama's quest to make the health care system accessible to all through government-backed health insurance is a point in question. Critics contend that this will bankrupt the economy because the health care industry is nonsustainable. Quality of medical care and access to services have sunk with the rise in health care insurance costs and in health 'management' systems where physicians' decisions are controlled by insurance agencies that put profit margins before patient care.

 With its emphasis on interventive rather than preventive and integrative medicine, and the escalating incidence of obesity, diabetes and a host of other disease which are preventable in the consumer populace, the health care system is clearly dysfunctional. The primary beneficiaries of any government funded health insurance scheme to enable people to access this health care system will be the pharmaceutical industry and a handful of CEOs and share holders. Secondary beneficiaries will be the petrochemical, agricultural and food industries, including the livestock and poultry industries with their cruel and disease spreading factory farms and feedlots.

 These industries continue to profit from nonsustainable, chemical- and drug-dependent methods of food production that put the health of millions of consumers in jeopardy. The widespread use of antibiotics by the livestock and poultry industries plays a significant role in the development of antibiotic resistant bacteria. The FDA estimates that two million people acquire bacterial infections in US hospitals annually, resulting in 90,000 deaths, 70 percent of which now involve bacteria resistant to at least one drug.

 The public pays for the production of basic food commodities (e.g. corn & soy) through billions of their annual tax dollars in the Farm Bill that allots subsidies that benefit these producers and commodity brokers.

Lowered costs for the food industry mean lower food prices in the market place for manufactured and processed foods and mass-produced animal products that the uneducated consumer accepts with out question, and under the erroneous belief that someone in government is really looking out for their well-being. The same must be said about most manufactured pet foods that result in otherwise preventable diseases in dogs and cats, many of which are shared by their owners, like cancer, immune system, neurological, developmental and endocrinological diseases like diabetes mellitus and hypothyroidism, as well as obesity, heart and kidney disease, and arthritis. According to US government reports, in 2009 two-thirds of the adult human population was overweight, and 34 percent were actually obese, while one-third of the child population is overweight with a shocking 17 percent obesity incidence. This is a mega-food-born epidemic that is quickly bankrupting the health care system, and undermines financial backing for educational, environmental, and employment-creation, with military employment and deployments escalating month by month, often coupled with US government and corporate funded foreign aid and disaster relief all subsidized by American citizens whose basic infrastructures are in dire need of repair and upgrading.

They also pay the price for deteriorating physical and mental health, which is in large measure products of what people eat and drink, medicate themselves with, and are prescribed. Except for selling dieting/weight reduction drugs, the pharmaceutical industry has profited royally from treating diabetics with insulin from millions of pigs—pharmaceutical 'pharming', that is now expanding as flocks and herds of genetically engineered animals are cloned to produce biological and medical products for the brave new animalpharm biotechnology industry.

While people's pets are like the proverbial canaries down the mineshaft, both humans and animals are the guinea pigs of a feeding experiment of unprecedented magnitude. It was so poorly designed that it is now almost impossible to monitor the safety of a new category of food ingredients that have been genetically engineered. These genetically modified (GM) ingredients are now in farmed animal feedstuffs, pet foods, and human foods, beverages, and various supplements. It was an earlier Republican administration that opened the market for the now global agricultural biotechnology industry with its patented varieties of GM crops from corn to soy. These are now the main ingredients used by the human, livestock and pet food industries—publicly subsidized no less—and their safety is now in question following several studies in laboratory animals that documented harmful effects on virtually all internal organs.

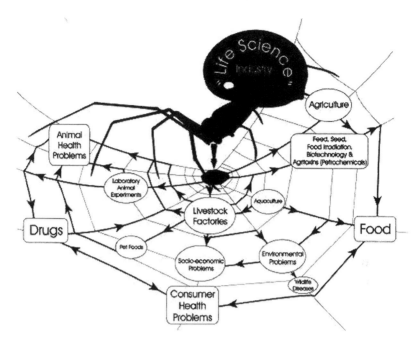

Figure 7-1. The Life Sciences Industry Web (from Bringing Life to Ethics, M.W. Fox, 2001)

The right solutions to health care reform are long overdue, and with clarity of vision, unclouded by ideology and by those vested interests hell bent on protecting the status quo of both the health care system and the food industry from censorship, accountability, and truth in advertising and labeling, there is hope for change. We should all follow the advice of Hippocrates, the founding father of modern medicine: 'Let your food be your medicine, and let your medicine be your food.'

CHAPTER 8
The Tripartite Nature of Integrative (Holistic) Medicine

The medical profession seems to have outdone the veterinary profession with a staggering incidence of adverse drug reactions (ADRs) in hospitalized patients. In one study, ADRs in the US ranked sixth in leading causes of death, with an estimated 2,216,000 ADRs, and 106,000 fatalities in hospitalized patients in 1994 (1). According to the FDA, 2 million people acquire bacterial infections while in hospital, and 90,000 die as a result. Alarmist as these figures may seem, they are symptomatic of the nemesis of modern medicine and of the urgent need for a more integrated, holistic approach to human illness that includes what we eat and how farmers farm (2).

The well-being of human patients' spirits is most often left to nurses and visiting clergy, and that of animal patients to veterinary nurses and caretakers, all of whom may or may not have the needed time, or sensitivity and training to fulfill this basic patient need. By well-being of spirit we mean, in the vernacular, subjective sense, as being in good spirits, as distinct from being dispirited.

Well-being in spirit is linked in part to the spiritual sensitivity, awareness, and depth of concern of healers and care-givers. Maximizing both should be an integral part of veterinary and human medical practice and teaching curricula. Attention to patients' well-being can be problematic for those who care but whose time is limited and treatments restricted due to the low reimbursements and dictates of seemingly one size fits all insurance directives.

Some veterinary practitioners have told me that they rigorously avoided having to hospitalize their patients because the adverse impact on animals' spirits was detrimental to recovery. They deplored some of their peers who over-hospitalized clients' animals, often for minor, ambulatory conditions for which more in-hospital tests and monitoring were advised.

The first duty is to make the patient as comfortable as possible by alleviating physical discomfort such as pain, and addressing compromising physiological states like fever and inflammation. Alleviation of fear, anxiety, agitation, and depression, all of which can aggravate physical signs of illness and compromise recovery, are also important responsibilities that good healers traditionally address.

The patient's vitality and condition of spirit have great prognostic value, since they are the manifest expression of the body-mind connection as evidenced in the patient's demeanor and changes therein during the course of the illness and treatment. The well-being of the spirit, an indicator of the will to live, is in part determined by physical and mental health. Sickness of the spirit, in extremis, the giving up of the will to live, has profound psychological and physiological consequences.

These concerns are gaining recognition today especially where elderly patients develop hospital psychosis or the hospitalism syndrome within a few days, becoming increasingly confused, disoriented, agitated, dispirited, anorexic, incontinent, and even hallucinatory. Comparable reactions may be seen in animals confined for treatment and either separated from their owners, regular care-takers, or from their own species-companions. Animals in some no-kill shelters become dispirited with inadequate human contact and environmental stimulation, becoming increasingly difficult to rehabilitate/re-socialize due to almost psychotic neophobia and fear of strangers. The cage-depression of such institutionalized animals, like those in poorly managed zoos and menageries, is often associated with stereotypic, obsessive-compulsive behaviors.

The well-being of the whole patient is addressed by the holistically oriented human and animal doctor who practices what I term integrated medicine. The cardinal signs of illness are closely evaluated, and diagnosis and treatment determined by considering the ways in which the illness in question is manifested. Physical and behavioral signs, called symptoms, may be treated directly, even in the absence of a formal diagnosis. Symptom-based treatments are supported by evidence-based medicine, drawing on prior experience with known remedies, not necessarily scientifically proven in terms of how the treatment actually works at the cellular level. When we, and the animals we care for, become ill, it is always for some reason, most often a multiplicity thereof. Elucidating the causes is half the cure, and the ultimate prevention.

The holistic healer intuitively senses and feels, through empathy, close observation, and communication with the patient, the condition of the spirit. Reasons for being dispirited are identified as well as possible, especially social and environmental influences, in addition to physical and mental factors. Of these there may be many that have a synergistic effect throughout every disease process that includes dis-ease, from the onset of symptoms to ultimate recovery or death.

Concern for the patient's spirit elevates medical and veterinary bioethics by incorporating values of compassion and empathy in patient treatment, care, and rehabilitation therapy. Decisions such as euthanasia, or discontinuing life-sustaining treatments, and evaluation of quality of life, can then be better made since the patient's quality of life and prognosis cannot always be determined on the basis of physical indices alone.

Conventional practitioners of allopathic animal and human medicine primarily base their healing practices on the use of various drugs (and surgeries). Western medical practice has separated the patient's body from the mind by obeying paradigms of a dualistic, mechanistic and reductionistic nature that have guided the approach to diagnosis and treatment. This has lead to some significant medical progress.

A further consequence has been the development of separate disciplines, beginning with psychiatry and internal medicine, and ending in oncology and dermatology, in part due to an exponential knowledge burden and demand for specialized skills. This development may contribute to the lack of conceptual and administrative integration, communication, and collaboration. The unforeseen sequelae of the birth of these specialized branches are breakdowns in public health and health-care services. The cost has been astronomical, despite miraculous breakthroughs in treatments and cures.

A similar breakdown secondary to this specialization-compartmentalization has been evolving in the veterinary profession. For example, some veterinary dermatology specialists and allergists, as well as general practitioners, fail to fully consider the role of manufactured pet foods in contributing to their patients' condition. Many over-prescribe steroid drugs, and even prescribe expensive manufactured 'prescription' diets that have been especially formulated ostensibly to treat various health problems from diabetes to dermatitis. Yet they often contain the very same food ingredients that were in the pet foods that caused or contributed to their patients' illness in the first place. (3)

Integrated Healing
Holistic veterinary and human doctors have gone beyond the false mind-body dichotomy in their approach to both diagnosis and treatment. The textbook edited by Dr. Frank McMillan entitled *Mental Health and Well-Being In Animals*,(4) and Schoen and Wynn's *Complementary and Alternative Veterinary Medicine*,(5) are part of this revolution/evolution of Western veterinary medicine toward an integrated approach in addressing animal health and disease prevention, and animal welfare and well-being.

One integrative approach is to encourage the ability to regard the patient's mind and body as his or her soul. One assumes that spirit is the animating principle of every living soul, whereby we will surely have a very different medical paradigm and approach to disease prevention and treatment. Once the separation of mind and body is rejected by conventional medical and veterinary practitioners, there is an opening for the integration of various alternative and supportive/adjunctive therapies.

Historically, the first breaking away from the dualistic dichotomy of psyche and soma came with the recognition of psychosomatic diseases in human patients, and subsequently in animal patients, (6). More recently, a major advance in integrative medicine has come with the recognition of epigenetic processes (7). These processes were inconceivable until the dualisms of organism and environment, genomes, nutrition and other prenatal influences, were overcome, along with the science-based fiction of genetic determinism.

My good friend, the late Professor Konrad Lorenz, MD, Nobel laureate and one of the founding fathers of ethology, once said, "Before you can really study an animal, you must first love it." By extension, before one can heal, one must first love the patient in the spiritual sense of agape. Within the clinical setting this means compassion and empathy, innate qualities rarely taught through example nor encouraged in either medical or veterinary schools, with a few recent exceptions. This is regrettable because most human-socialized animals, like children, sense when they are loved, and whether someone is genuine or not. As with pediatricians, veterinarians who feign affection for their patients do not get very far.

The science of ethology helps resolve the artificial mind-body duality since it provides the tools to objectively determine the highly subjective condition of the animal's ethos, its spirit, sentiment, character, or disposition. The addition of applied animal ethology to the veterinary teaching curriculum has done much to dispel the long-held view that animals do not have feelings, cannot suffer psychologically or become dispirited.

The collective ethos of society in terms of how animals are perceived and ought to be treated has changed significantly over the past 3-4 decades. Humane concerns are being raised about how and why animals are being treated in certain ways. The veterinary profession is being called upon by society to address many of these concerns as they affect animals' health and well-being. In the eyes of some critics, the profession has taken more reactive and defensive roles than proactive initiatives in order to protect the vested interests of their animal industry and commercial clients. This conventional view has deep cultural roots. The veterinary, medical, and medical research disciplines need to disentangle themselves from such corporate entities. They must refocus conceptually, perceptually, ideologically, and ethically on animal health and well-being for animals' sake as well as for the public health and other community benefits.

The cultural blindness toward animals as living souls who are sentient beings is still very much in evidence today, reflected in the dispirited eyes of self-mutilating primates and purpose-bred dogs who spend most if not all of their lives in small laboratory cages or pens; in the eyes of arthritis-crippled breeding sows in factory farms who are so confined as to be unable to walk or turn around their entire lives; and in the eyes of performing circus elephants who spend most of their lives in chains and usually die from chronic foot infections and osteomyelitis.

The inability of animals to express their ethos, the normal range of behaviors essential for their physical and psychological well-being, because of the conditions under which we keep them, is to deny them expression of their natures, their spirits. To what ends and to what degree we chose to inhibit, even crush their spirits, is a bioethical issue that society has yet to fully address. But, along with the veterinary profession, society cannot address this issue with impartial objectivity until the chauvinistic notion of human superiority that puts people before other animals is tempered by humility and equalitarianism—giving all sentient beings equally fair consideration.

Charles Darwin asserted that "The difference in mind between man and higher animals, great as it is, certainly is one of degree and not of kind." (8). He wrote these words over a century ago, contrary to the prevailing anthropocentrism of the time, based upon his studies of comparative morphology and behavior. In a similar vein, the late Loren Eiseley, a professor of anthropology and paleontology, (9) observed, "One does not meet oneself until one catches the reflection from an eye other than human." Such self-discovery would do much, I believe, to improve the

health and well-being of our own kind, and the animals under our care.
Now to revisit some of the issues raised in earlier chapters with a more in-depth consideration of agricultural practices and the products of the global food industry, including genetically engineered crops and manufactured pet foods, many of which veterinarians are selling and which at this time of writing contribute to a host of health problems in dogs and especially cats. As will be revealed, some of these diet-related problems are shared by people whose food choices are ill informed by taste/palatability (sweet, salty and fatty), and by a constant barrage of fast and convenience food advertisements and special discounts.

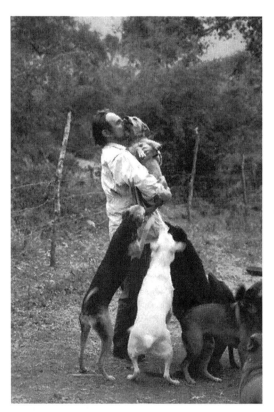

Figure 8-1. A canine love pyramid greets Dr Fox as he holds Dean, the pack leader, at Deanna Krantz's animal refuge in South India (Photograph by India Project for Animals & Nature)

CHAPTER 9
Agriculture or Agricide & the Global FDA Food-Drug & Agribusiness Complex

'Who ever could make two ears of corn or two blades of grass
to grow up on a spot of ground where only one grew before
would deserve better of mankind and do more essential service
to his country than the whole race of politicians put together.'—
Jonathan Swift, 1667-1745. Irish-born priest and writer.

"The significant problems of the world cannot be solved at the same level
of consciousness at which they were created."—Albert Einstein

Summary
Food safety, quality and security are rising concerns both nationally and
internationally. The hegemony of multinational agribusiness corporations
promoting nonsustainable agricultural practices erodes both cultural
and biological diversity; promotes cruel and environmentally damaging
concentrated animal feeding operations (CAFOs or factory farms)
supported by wholesale use of antibiotics, anabolic steroids, live vaccines,
pesticides, and other veterinary drugs; and the planting of patented,
genetically engineered/modified (GM) and hybrid crop varieties coupled
with toxic agrichemical pesticides and fertilizers.
    The validity of these concerns will be documented from a holistic
veterinary, public and environmental health perspective. The bioethical
basis for the adoption of bioregionally appropriate, sustainable, community
supported and supporting, socially just, humane, and organically certified
farming practices and marketing cooperatives will be established. In
the face of climate change, rising oil and food prices, dwindling food
reserves, and increasing world hunger, finding and applying alternatives to
conventional, petrochemical-based agribusiness is one of humanity's most
urgent priorities.

The Transnational FDA

The late President of the United States, Dwight Eisenhower cautioned, 'Beware of the industrial-military complex.' In today's global context, the transnational FDA (food, drug and agribusiness) industrial complex needs to be confronted and dismantled.

Poverty and hunger are exacerbated by the disenfranchisement of indigenous farmers and once sustainable communities by commodity crop developments and subsidized imports, including crops grown to feed livestock and poultry for the more affluent urban consumers. Landless 'peasants' become the urban poor, their indigenous wisdom, sustainable farming systems, and crop and livestock varieties being lost in the process.

The harmful socioeconomic consequences of so called CAFOs (concentrated animal feeding operations, i.e. bio-concentration camps/ factory farms) in the US have been well documented. Once independent family farms have become extinct, either forced into bankruptcy or contracted into corporate serfdom by large, and increasingly transnational agribusiness conglomerates.

The global imperialism of such monopolists is assured when tax payer's moneys go to heavily subsidize commodity crops and animal feedstuffs. These farm subsidies help this agribusiness sector gain an advantage in the competitive world market place, but much to the detriment of America's once vibrant and productive nexus of family farms and rural communities, now decimated by this juggernaut of economism that is called progress and necessity. Trade agreements through NAFTA and the WTO, (the North American Free Trade Association and the World Trade Organization), with their transnational laws and regulations set up to facilitate the fixing of prices, supply, and demand, violate the sovereignty of nation states and the viability of farming communities world-wide.

Conditioned Chemical & Drug Addictions

We are all conditioned as children to take our medicine, and as adults to trust the good doctor and not question Aesculapian authority. In science we all trust. Anything that is called 'scientific' or 'science-based' is acceptable. But Aesculapian authority needs to be questioned, and the pharmaceutical industry held accountable for violating public trust with its rush to fast-track new drugs and vaccines for government approval, patent protection and world-market profits. Agribusiness' petrochemical industry claims scientific authority over the 'safe and effective' application of pesticides— agricidal poisons— to the land as well as to the food-chains of man and beast. This same industry lobbies against any restrictions on the use of antibiotics in livestock feed, and other food-animal veterinary biologics/ drugs that substitute for more humane, disease-preventing methods of livestock and poultry production; putting both humans and animals at risk in the process.

The food and drug industry complex with its pharmaceutical and petrochemical and 'life science' agribiotechnology components is not to be trusted. The public trust has been violated in countless ways in the rush for corporate profits and market monopolies. How can we trust the medical profession that condones the wholesale medication of even kindergarten children, with psychotropic, mood and behavior-altering pharmaceuticals? Or organized veterinary medicine that never opposed the use of antibiotics as feed-additive growth-stimulants for poultry and livestock? Neither the American Medical nor Veterinary Medical Associations opposed government approval BGH—genetically engineered bovine growth hormone—the first product of animal production biotechnology to be rushed to market, before the rash of genetically modified live virus vaccines. (BGH is prohibited in Canada and the UK for cow heath and public health reasons). Who can trust the food industry when it is public knowledge that the 'life science' biotechnology industry-government alliance allowed the planting and consumption of never-tested or authorized, yet patented (even by the US government) varieties of genetically engineered food and feed crops? (See Chapter 11 for documented concerns). The enduring government alliance with the petrochemical pesticide and fertilizer companies that continue to poison our food and water, and contaminate our oceans and amniotic fluids, with all the drugs consumed that we and livestock excrete, is a matter of fact.

Profits and pestilence aside, the veterinary and human medical advocates of conventional vaccines and drugs for a sickening society and sickly, stressed factory farmed livestock and poultry, can no longer ignore the price of success: Nor can the agribusiness food industry, squandering land, water and oil/fossil fuels to boost production and profits with its toxic petrochemical fertilizers and pesticides.

Drugs & Farm Animal Health

CAFOs (concentrated animal feeding operations or 'factory' farms) are a bad investment in the long-term. Notably, they are pathogenic, spreading agricologenic and domestogenic diseases—new crop and animal pathogens and the chronic human diseases associated with the Western diet. They are also a major source of diseases of food-born origin, often epidemic in scale, and other diseases like Avian and Swine 'flu. New zoonotic diseases, and more virulent strains of existing zoonotic pathogens, are likely to evolve because of the pathogenic environments and condition of the animals incarcerated in CAFOs.

Like agrichemicals, not all vaccines are bad. But like many drugs they stimulate populations of pathogens and harmless organisms to mutate and become more harmful. So we need new, more costly— and highly profitable—mutation and serovar-specific vaccines and ever stronger antibiotics and other drugs. The same is true with the application of agricultural, food industry pesticides, a global industry, along with genetically engineered crops, that stimulate populations of resistant weeds, insect pest, and crop diseases. And both human and veterinary drugs and agrichemicals cause serious water contamination.

Human and veterinary vaccines and drugs give us a false sense of security and put us on the treadmill of addiction/dependency to prevent and treat diseases in essentially pathogenic environments, notably those where there is human over-crowding, poverty and malnutrition, and where virtually genetically homozygous farmed animals are crowded together in CAFOs, mirroring the genetic uniformity of commodity crops grown in disease-promoting monocultures.

Ideal substrates/environments for the proliferation of pathogens have been created in CAFOs with the commercial hybrid livestock and poultry lines being virtually homozygous—and now even being cloned. This calls for more drugs and vaccines—what I call domestogenic diseases of animal production—that mirror the agricologenic pest and blight problems of crops that are also raised in homozygotic (genetically uniform) monocultures on nutrient-and micro-organism deficient, agrichemically intoxicated soils.

Factory farmed animals are made genetically as uniform as possible in terms of growth rates/productivity, in order to maximize profits. Genetic uniformity is even more so when they have been cloned, a biogenetic engineering process now in full swing. Genetically similar lines of pigs for example, make similar weight gains and reach slaughter weight at the same time. This uniformity mirrors that of commodity food and feed crops grown in monocultures. Both provide ideal substrates/environments for the proliferation and evolution of increasingly virulent and highly infectious and contagious organisms. Coupled with husbandry factors such as over-crowding stress, soil nutrient deficiencies etc; this lack of genetic diversity increases the virulence of organisms, even making harmless ones, (so called commensals and symbiotes) into pathogens and pests. Those pathogens that can rapidly mutate or acquire genetic material from other organisms can soon develop resistance to antibiotics, pesticides, and other drugs, in some instances even thriving on them.

Deliberately infecting already immuno-compromised animals in CAFOs with modified /attenuated, yet still live viral vaccines is problematic and counter-intuitive considering the zoonotic, public health risks, manufacturers' profits notwithstanding. The various antibiotics, anti-parasite, and other veterinary drug residues, including anabolic steroids and growth hormone implants, and feed additives and contaminants like copper, arsenic, cadmium, lead and dioxin that go into the environment in animals' nitrogenous and phosphate-loaded excrement, pose a challenging management and containment problem, (especially to surface and ground water) that few if any CAFOs effectively address.

Recycling slaughtered livestock and poultry remains along with food and beverage industry by-products into livestock and poultry feeds which are not organically certified and therefore can contain pesticide residues as well as dioxins, heavy metals, and various pathogens, can seriously compromise animal health and welfare. Manufactured livestock and poultry diets can be deficient in essential nutrients, and being formulated to increase growth/productivity at the lowest possible ingredient cost to maximize profits, can result in production-related diseases, notably metabolic and liver diseases in cattle, arthritis/lameness in pigs, and lameness, obesity and heart attacks in broiler chickens. . Feeding livestock and poultry GM herbicide and insect resistant crops and byproducts containing endogenous toxins like Bt, and absorbed herbicides, and conventional feed from nutrient deficient soils and hybrid 'Green Revolution' crop varieties, pose further animal and consumer health issues.

One of the most limiting factors in establishing CAFOs is the diminishing supply of water world-wide, and the vast quantities demanded by such operations. The amount of land and resources used to raise feed and fodder for intensively raised, confined livestock and poultry has a major impact on biodiversity. The negative impact on wildlife habitat is compounded by the adverse wildlife and habitat impacts of extensive livestock husbandry systems of grazing/ ranching/ pastoralism where there is over-stocking/over-grazing, and indiscriminate predator control. The adoption of sustainable livestock production systems linked with organic food, feed and fodder production appropriate to the natural resource availability in given bioregions would do much to help advance the conservation-based agriculture approach to wildlife protection and habitat restoration.

Farm Animal Health & Welfare Concerns

Because it stood by and did nothing other than eagerly offer professional advice and services, organized veterinary medicine in most all industrialized countries is in large part responsible for the suffering of billions of intensively raised farm animals on so called factory farmed and feedlots. Farmed animal health, behavioral and welfare issues associated with these food animal production methods, (now referred to by the industry as confinement animal feeding operations or CAFOs), were seen as a challenge rather than as symptoms of husbandry systems and practices that were bioethically unacceptable and should never exist. But they soon spread to developing countries under the support of agencies like the World Bank and British Overseas Development Corporation which are linked with multinational agribusiness interests, from livestock feed drugs and vaccines to breeding stock and vertically integrated market monopolies.

I have visited these animal concentration camps and documented the suffering, stress and distress of poultry, pigs and cattle, including dairy cows, beef cattle and veal calves under conditions that deprive them of their basic behavioral needs and of any quality of life, all in the name of profit and 'production efficiencies' that are touted as reducing consumer costs.

It took over 25 years since the publication of my book *Farm Animals: Husbandry, Behavior and Veterinary Practice* (Baltimore, Maryland, University Park Press, 1984), along with the reports by others documenting the connections between CAFOs, animal diseases and related public health and environmental concerns for the World Health Organization, the Food and Agriculture Organization and the World Organization for Animal Health to acknowledge these connections and to begin to work together to find solutions. (See www.oie.int/eng/press/en_100422.htm). Organized veterinary medicine in Europe and North America has begun to rally (too little too late?), one editorial in the *British Veterinary Record*, (June 5th, 2010, p 702) noting "The concept of 'one world, one health, one medicine' has so much to commend it that it is surprising that it has not caught on more quickly." I find it not surprising considering the denial of the evils of CAFOs and the gulling of consumers into believing that this is the way modern farming is done to make food affordable and to feed the hungry world.

Such unconscionable mistreatment of sentient beings is a sad reflection of our own lack of humanity which cannot be justified even if these animals were bred and raised simply for human consumption and knew no better life prior to their slaughter. It underscores the truism that when we harm others we harm ourselves.

The following is a brief synopsis of the major health and welfare concerns that can only be rectified not by strict 'humane' standards, inspections and enforcement, but by the phasing out of all such methods of animal production, and the adoption of husbandry systems that provide for animals' physical and behavioral needs and that are ecologically integrated with sustainable farming practices.

Farm Animal Health & Welfare Concerns: Synopsis

All the below concentrated animal feeding operations cause stress, distress, and increased disease susceptibility especially to enteric and respiratory infections, and to udder/mammary gland infections in dairy cows.

- Caged Laying Hens: Extreme overcrowding, lack of movement induced osteoporosis, bone fractures, foot lesions from wire floor, feather-picking, and cannibalism.
- Broiler Chickens: Extreme overcrowding, lameness, contact dermatitis (breast blisters), ascites, (dropsy), feather picking and cannibalism, 'keel-over' heart-failure from rapid growth. Eye problems, including blindness, from poor ventilation. Constant hunger due to food restriction of breeding stock.
- Penned Piglets: Overcrowding, boredom, tail-biting, cannibalism, lameness and foot lesions from a life on concrete slatted floors. Circulation and joint problems from rapid growth and large body mass: Chronic respiratory problems from poor ventilation.
- Breeding Sows in crates: Extreme physical constraint (unable to walk or turn around), lameness, arthritis, boredom and stereotypic behaviors indicative of stress and distress.
- Veal Calves in crates: Extreme physical constraint, (unable to walk or turn around), social deprivation, iron-deficient diet causing anemia and weakness.
- Feedlot Beef Cattle: Exposure-lack of shade and shelter, lameness and foot rot, liver disease from improper 'fattening/finishing' diets and lack of roughage.
- Confined Dairy Cows: lack of exercise related lameness, metabolic, and liver diseases from high energy/concentrate diets and lack of roughage.

The following procedures need to be addressed and where appropriate, either phased out, or only the most humane methods permitted:

Castrating, branding, and dehorning cattle without anesthetic; hot-iron de-beaking of chickens; disposal of unwanted chickens & pre-slaughter collecting and handling of poultry; tail docking and castration of piglets and lambs; tail docking of dairy cows; treatment of unwanted 'bobby' calves and 'downer cows;' and of sick and injured poultry and piglets. Use of the 'Stock-still' electrical immobilization of cattle should be prohibited. Humane methods for the mass 'depopulating/killing of diseased livestock and poultry also need to be implemented.

Livestock and poultry transportation, handling, and slaughter methods need significant improvements in most counties.

Population & Consumption Issues

The price of success in maintaining and promoting human population growth with decreased mortality rates and arguably longer life expectancies means more hungry mouths to feed and potential disease outbreaks to fend off. In more affluent and consumptive socioeconomic sectors around the world the diseases of affluence like obesity-diabetes/metabolic syndrome, and cancer, are part of the price of success. But the ever more impoverished and landless survivors of averted epidemics and famines, and the more affluent but disenchanted, together make the kindling of inter-tribal conflicts, war and acts of terrorism inevitable.

Uncoupled from any family planning and concerted population control, effective resource management and conservation, pollution control, sustainable agricultural practices and economies local and global, poverty, sickness and famine will be the legacy of the human condition, passed on with increasing virulence from one generation to the next. Look at our history since the beginning of the Industrial Revolution, the Age of Reason, and the epoch of colonial imperialism, once nationalistic, now corporate and transnational. The fear- based progress and the success of the modern age envisioned by the military-industrial technocracy generations ago, to essentially find ways to profit in the name of fighting famine and pestilence, two of our primal fears, by selling more drugs to save more people—for what? And by selling more toxic chemicals to produce more food—for why, but mainly to fatten the cattle of the rich as Gandhi observed, now mean that there are ever more mouths to feed and souls to suffer.

The price of success in maintaining unhealthy concentrations of animals for human consumption and for other commercial purposes, made possible by the use of veterinary vaccines, antibiotics and other drugs, has meant more resistant and harmful pathogens, more and more being

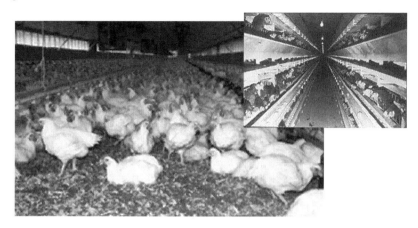

Figure 9-1. Broiler chickens in Shed (Battery-caged laying hens above)

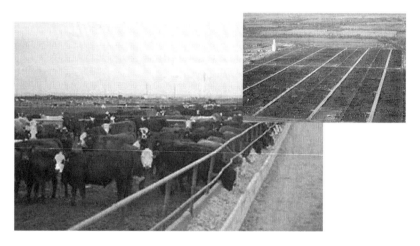

Figure 9-2. Beef Cattle feed Lot (Aerial of feed lots above)

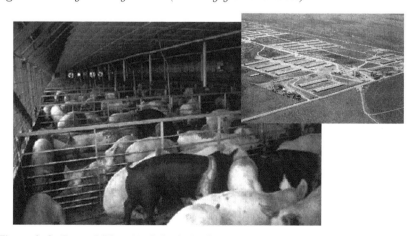

Figure 9-3. Penned Pigs (Aerial of pig farm above. Photographs by M.W. Fox)

harmful to humans, the so-called zoonotic diseases. When computed along with the environmental impact of extensive livestock herding and grazing, CAFOs are a major contributor to climate change; and a leader of the pack in ground and surface water pollution and topsoil waste.

Corporate profits notwithstanding, the misguided altruism of philanthropic agencies and individuals playing into the FDA system, giving $ billions in drugs, food aid, and seed and livestock varieties unsuited for sustainable farming, is a major impediment to real progress in the human condition that is inseparable from environmental health and quality, and from the protection and restoration of both cultural and biological diversity.

Western Diet & Health

It is argued that without the use of the petrochemical industry's fuel, pesticides and fertilizers, and the genetically engineered commodity crops of its agribiotechnology affiliates, commercial, high-volume crops like cotton, corn and soy could never be produced in the amount that is needed to clothe and to feed people ever more beef and cheese, rather than whole wheat and organic rye, and more pork and chicken rather than lentils and beans. The Western economy, and the middle class in particular that has been raised on this diet (of the affluent), rather than on the healthier, organic, minimally processed cereal/grain, legume, fruit and vegetable-based diets of the materially poorer indigenous peoples around much of the world, are being crushed by the rising drug and health care costs, primarily arising from a meat and processed 'junk' food- based diet. While informed Westerners adopt some of the more healthful diets of indigenous peoples, their own governments, and donor, 'philanthropic' agencies, like the UN's World Bank, are working to implant their own industrial agriculture and the Western diet in developing countries to sate the rising demands of the affluent, and the tourist industry, for beef, chicken, cheese, ice cream, and in non-Muslim countries, more pork instead of lentils, chick peas and beans.

The irony that the Western diet is now being associated with not only such epidemic problems as obesity, stroke, heart attack, diabetes and chronic degenerative diseases like arthritis as well as a range of cancers and birth defects and brain damage, but also with behavioral changes in the consumer populace. Most notable is the epidemic incidence of anxiety and obsessive compulsive, addictive, and depressive disorders, and various psychoses, violent and delusional. These behavioral abnormalities are associated with disrupted brain, neuroendocrine system chemistry, like the neurochemicals serotonin and nor-adrenaline. While social and emotional stress contribute to these complex and widespread mental health problems, radical dietary changes that are the antithesis of the Western diet and that embrace some of the nutritional wisdom of earlier times and indigenous traditions, have been shown to greatly help many of these neurobehavioral, psychological, and psychosomatic disorders, especially in children.

We may never know to what degree we have harmed ourselves, even for ever, genetically, with petrochemical pesticides that are lipophilic, being selectively absorbed by fatty tissues, as in the skin of oranges, the breasts of women, and the brains of all.

More and more people, along with their pets, make dramatic recoveries from a variety of health problems following a change in diet that includes the exclusion of almost all the conventional human and companion animal (cat and dog) prepared and processed foods.

That highly refined, denatured, and bleached wheat flour was sold as 'Wonder Bread' for decades in the US, while the more nutritious ingredients were either put into livestock feed, or used by other food industry sectors, including the 'health food' industry that sold at premium prices the bran, gluten and vitamins that was taken out of Wonder Bread, as essential dietary supplements. Wonder Bread is the Asian and Middle and Far Eastern equivalent of polished white rice, the essentially denatured, nutritionally deficient staple food of billions of uninformed people.

Much of the food we consume today and that goes in to pet foods and livestock feed are from 'high performance' patented hybrid seed varieties that were developed in the 1960's and '70's as part of the much hyped 'Green Revolution' to feed the hungry world and end famine and malnutrition around the globe.

'Green Revolution' Harms & Costs
In the 1990 declaration by the International Movement for Ecological Agriculture meeting in Penang, Malaysia, the following critical comments were made on the Green Revolution:

'Modern intensive agriculture has conspicuously failed to increase food production and to meet global food and nutrition needs. The claim that the Green Revolution has led to higher crop yields is highly exaggerated and does not reflect a fair and complex comparison with more ecologically sound systems:

These claims are usually based on the measurement of yield as defined per acre or hectare of land. However, if one takes into account the hidden costs on input subsidies and nonrenewable resources, and the costs of ecological damage (leading to lower yields after some time) and furthermore, measure yield against high fertilizer and water costs, then the Green Revolution techniques are highly inefficient. In contrast, the economic soundness is striking of traditional and ecologically better varieties.

Even more seriously, the Green Revolution measurement of output is flawed because it only accounts for a single crop (e.g., rice) and even then only a single component of that crop (e.g., grain) whilst neglecting the uses of straw for fodder and fertilizer. Thus, it neglects to take into account that there were many other biological resources (e.g., other crops, other no-grain uses of the measured crop and fish) within the same land in the traditional system that were reduced or wiped out with the Green Revolution. If output is measured in terms of total biomass, a more realistic picture of the performance of the Green Revolution will emerge.

Although yields of food crops in total have increased, less food is available to local populations. There are several reasons for this: There has been an increase in a few cereals (a large volume of which is fed to cattle in the North) at the expense of pulses and other crops; The increased dependency of Third World farmers and countries on intensive inputs has led to indebtedness and the breakdown of self-sufficiency; Much of the increased food production is exported, thus denying the food to local people; Many areas planted with high-yielding varieties (which are actually high-response varieties to the applied inputs, including chemical fertilizers and pesticides) are now experiencing diminishing returns; Ecological degradation is leading to reduced yields and to the abandonment of many areas of agricultural land; Losses during storage have increased markedly in many areas; The low prices paid for farm produce and the high prices charged for food in the shops, combined with increased levels of indebtedness, ensure that many farmers cannot afford to buy sufficient food for their families.'

(END OF DECLARATION)

The failure of the Green Revolution was underscored in a report from the UK's Global Environmental Change Programme, funded by Britain's Economic and Research Council, and published in April 2000.Green Revolution crops, introduced in the late 1960's and early 1970's increased agricultural output and profits, and provided much needed and affordable calories for the poor. But these crops failed to take up minerals such as iron and zinc from the soil. The report states: "High yielding Green Revolution crops were introduced in poor countries to overcome famine. But these are now blamed for causing intellectual deficits, because they do not take up essential micronutrients." Iron deficiency disease contributes to increased infant mortality, impaired brain development and learning ability, affecting an estimated 1.5 billion people in one quarter of the earth's population, according to the author of this report, Dr. Christopher Williams.

It should also be added that micronutrient deficiencies, also a nutritional problem in the West from deficient soils and crops, can impair the immune system, and related nutritional deficiencies and imbalances in various animal products, especially in the omega 3and 6 polyunsaturated fatty acid ratios can impair brain development and cognitive functions. Recent studies in Canada, the U. S. and the U. K. have shown that fruits and vegetables are less nutritious than 30-50 years ago, showing often marked deficiencies in iron, copper, zinc, calcium, sodium, phosphorus, protein, vitamins C and riboflavin, a disturbing finding attributable, in part, to the fast-growing and large-yielding varieties of crops being grown today for human consumption: And to the use of chemical fertilizers, potassium fertilizer, for example, interferes with plants' magnesium and phosphate absorption. Herbicides like Monsanto's Roundup can interfere with plants' uptake of iron and manganese. Widely used nitrogenous fertilizers can increase harmful nitrate levels in conventionally grown crops, lower the plant's vitamin C content, and while increasing total protein content, the quality of the protein is inferior to organically grown crops, lacking in essential amino acids like lysine, which means lower quality food, and livestock feed.

Organic is Superior

Studies comparing the nutrient content of organic versus conventionally grown crops report significantly lower levels of potentially toxic aluminum, mercury and lead in the organically grown, that also had higher levels of many essential trace minerals and other nutrients, notably boron, calcium, chromium, copper, iodine, iron, lithium, magnesium, manganese, molybdenum, phosphorus, potassium, selenium, silicon, sodium, sulfur, vanadium, and zinc. Also more vitamin C, bioflavonoids and other antioxidants, and less nitrate. Produce from animals fed organically grown feed are more nutritious than from CAFO raised animals fed manufactured food-and beverage industry byproducts and synthetic supplements and drugs. Organic beef has more healthful Omega 3; organic chicken has more Vitamin E, Omega 3 and beta carotene; organic milk has more antioxidants, lutein and zeanthine.

Animal studies have shown that such functions as reproduction and resistance to infection may be adversely affected by conventionally produced foods as compared to organically produced ones.

Studies around the world of organic farming methods found that they contributed more to biodiversity and wildlife conservation than do more harmful conventional farming practices .Organic agriculture increases biodiversity at every level of the food chain, from soil bacteria to wild mammals and raptors.

University of Michigan professors Catherine Badgley and Ivette Perfecto have completed a three-year study of worldwide organic vs. conventional farm yields and found that organic farming could produce three times as much as low-intensive methods on the same farms in developing countries, and to produce almost equal yields to conventional farms in developed countries.

Like holistic medicine, organic farming is systemically integrated within the physical parameters of general systems theory and quantum mechanics as they relate to dynamic living ecosystems, with the overlays of ethics, esthetics, and metaphysics. As 2008 President of the Pennsylvania Sustainable Agriculture Association's annual conference, dairy farmer Kim Seeley advised in his opening address, that we must all "Obey Nature's laws first before we accept man's laws."

That more holistically-oriented physicians, veterinarians, and agronomists are at last beginning to put such wisdom in to practice is a clear sign that a paradigm shift or change in our worldview is taking place and that the status-quo of conventional medicine, agriculture, the economy, and other social institutions is no longer acceptable and most certainly not viable without further violence and suffering. As more medical and veterinary scientists are becoming real healers, so more farmers are becoming real land-stewards.

Their paradigm is based upon the following bioethical principles: compassion, service, humility, ahimsa (avoiding causing harm), and reverential respect for all life; social justice; eco-justice, and the precautionary principle. These are the cornerstones of a healthy community and of a sustainable economy. We have all but eliminated the Meadowlark from our fields. We have many wrongs to right, and much to atone for what our ancestors and civilization have done to harm through fear and ignorance, arrogance and greed.

Advances in the science and bioethics of alternative human and veterinary medicine and organic agriculture that are based on this new paradigm hold much promise and should be supported by the corporate sector as well as by the consumer-populace and their governments.

Reducing Animal Consumption: A Bioethical Imperative
The singularly most damaging environmental footprint upon this planet is caused by our collectively costly and damaging appetite for meat. Some 3.2 billion cattle, sheep and goats are now being raised for human consumption, along with billions more pigs and poultry. These extensively

and intensively farmed animals produce less food for us than they consume, and compete with us for water. Their numbers and appetites result in an increasing loss wildlife and habitat, and of good farmlands and grazing lands. Linked with deforestation, loss of wetlands, over-fishing and ocean pollution, our appetite for meat is the number one cause of global warming/climate change.

We can no longer continue to regard meat and other sources of animal protein as a dietary staple because of the enormous costs and harmful consequences of such a diet. Vegetarianism is an enlightened choice, and all people should at least become 'conscientious omnivores,' treating food of animal origin more as a condiment than a staple. According to figures from the UK's Compassion in World Farming, reported in The Economist (Dec. 2nd 2006, p. 88) over 50 billion animals are killed for food every year, which comes to almost 100,000 a minute 24/7. In the past 40 year meat consumption per person has risen from 56 kg to 89 in Europe, from 89 kg to 124 in America, and from 4 kg to 54 in China, in spite of the nutritionally inefficient conversion of grass or grain to meat, some 10 kg of feed being needed to produce 1 kg of meat.

It is surely a bioethical imperative not to kill animals for their flesh when no less nutritious foods of plant origin are readily available, more affordable, and more sustainably produced. Ironically, the shift toward 'improved' animal-based diet correlates with increased incidence of so called Western diseases, and with an increasingly dysfunctional, unhealthy environment.

These correlations support the karmic truism that when we harm others—animals and the natural environment—we harm ourselves. Hence obedience to the Golden Rule—of treating others as we would have them treat us, is enlightened self interest. This core bioethical principle is embraced by the animal rights and environmental/deep ecology movements that have been demonized by antidisestablishmentarians who have succeeded with the Bush administration to identify both movements as potential terrorist organizations liable for prosecution under the Bioterrorism Preparedness Act of 2002. Homeland Security and the protection of vested interests are one and the same, the continued, economically justified exploitation and suffering of animals, and environmental desecration, being protected under the law. U.S. animal industries have gained additional protection with the so called Animal Enterprise Protection Act that criminalizes certain conduct aimed against companies engaged in animal production, research and testing.

The economy of the Western industrial consumerist paradigm

is nonsustainable, and because of its global reach, is wreaking global havoc, as predicted by Jared Diamond and many other visionaries and critics of these times. For instance, much livestock feed is imported by the multinational food industry oligopolists from the impoverished third world, thus contributing to mass malnutrition in poorer countries. This problem is compounded by what is called 'dumping' of surplus, heavily subsidized, animal and other agricultural products/commodities on the third world, from chicken legs and powdered milk, to corn and wheat, often under the guise of emergency food aid. This only serves to enrich a corrupt few, and undermines the economic viability of indigenous farmers and once sustainable rural communities.

In sum, we can no longer continue to regard meat and other sources of animal protein as a dietary staple because of the enormous costs and harmful consequences of such a diet. Vegetarianism is an enlightened choice, and all people should at least become 'conscientious omnivores,' treating food of animal origin more as a condiment than as a staple.

Beware of the FDA's 'Life Science'

Industrial agribusiness' indifference and corpus of denial of toward the suffering of intensively raised farm animals parallels the indifference toward all the harmful agrichemical pesticides and fertilizers that are now in our rain, food, drinking water, mothers' milk, and even amniotic fluids, and that have turned the countryside into a toxic chemical wasteland.

The infamy and hegemony of the multinational, oligopolistic corporations like Monsanto, Novartis, and Syngenta, that have named their business the 'Life Science' industry, pushing these agricultural inputs from seed and equipment to chemical fertilizers and pesticides onto developing countries, after decimating the once sustainable network of small farming and food processing operations in the Americas and Europe, and much of the rest of the industrial, 'developed' world, are a matter of public, historic record. This multinational industry essentially 'out-sources' agricultural production of commodity crops that it imports to the US on the cheap from countries where poverty and corruption often rampant, and where agricultural chemicals banned in the US are widely used.

A major, global venture of this Life Science industry has been to develop varieties of high-yield hybrid seeds, and more recently, genetically engineered seeds that are resistant to herbicides, produce their own pesticides, nutrient supplements for livestock, (like lysine that factory farmed pigs need a lot of), and even pharmaceutical drugs, created not to feed the hungry world, but for patent-protected, new and profitable commodities. During the 1980's these monopoly players—the petrochemical, pharmaceutical and life science conglomerates—rushed to buy up all independent seed companies and their seed stocks. Patented, high yield hybrid varieties are few in number, widely planted, and genetically uniform. The uniformity means genetic vulnerability to disease (same for the patented hybrid strains of commercially farmed animals). It is these highly inbred, hybrid varieties that are now being genetically engineered, and spreading worldwide at the ever quickening pace of global monopoly.

The seed stocks of conventional and heirloom varieties are not being planted, are deteriorating in storage, and when planted are likely to become contaminated by the pollen of genetically engineered crops from neighboring fields and counties. This accelerating decline in the genetic diversity of our major food, feed and fiber (and biomass and green manure) crops, coupled with the genetic disruption of plant genomes that the genetic engineering process can cause (see Chapter 11) call for a total moratorium on any further plantings of GM seeds. As referenced below, there are enough documented research studies to negate the government-industry response to such a moratorium and community-linked GM-FREE Zones that would say that there is no scientific evidence of harm to animals or to human consumers, and that GM seeds are 'substantially equivalent' to conventional varieties.

The socially and politically disruptive and devastating human suffering soon to come, according to some agronomists, including Nobel laureate Norman Borlaug (whose crop 'improvement' genetic research has arguably caused more harm than good in the hands of agribusiness oligopolies) is from the Ug99 strain of black stem rust fungus on the world's wheat crop. This world wheat crop has so little genetic diversity now that there are few varieties and cultivars with any genetic resistance to this devastating disease that could mean global famine. Putting all our eggs in the same basket is never a wise investment.

This Life Science industry has convinced legislators that genetically engineered crops are safe, and 'substantially equivalent' to conventional varieties of food and animal feed crops. But the scientific evidence, and documented animal safety tests, point in the opposite direction. The US government even attempted to have genetically engineered seeds and foods included under the National Organic Standards. Genetically engineered crops of corn, soy and canola that are herbicide resistant, and corn that produces its own insecticidal poison called Bt, get into the human food chain, and are put into livestock feed and pet foods with the government's blessing: And quite probably to the demise of the honey bee and a large agricultural sector of bee-pollination dependent orchard and field crops.

Herbicide resistant crops actually absorb the herbicide that is repeatedly sprayed to kill competing weeds which we and the animals subsequently consume, along with whatever endogenous pesticides they have been genetically engineered to produce and have been treated with from seed to shelf.

As for the documented, peer-reviewed, published studies generally mandated by good judgment before the government's approving any novel food, such as a genetically engineered one, there were virtually none made public before and after the Life Science Industry developed and patented new GM foods and animal feeds and put them on the market. In spite of worldwide public opposition, GM crops and seeds have respectively come to dominate and contaminate both conventional and organic food and industrial commodity crop markets.

The oil-shortage panic move in the U.S to ill advised ethanol production from corn will mean more plantings of GM varieties, less land for livestock feed, and for human food-crop production to stockpile for humanitarian emergency relief food programs that are in more demand than ever with climate change.

Arguably the worst case scenario of nonsustainable industrial agriculture is the U.S. government's commodity crop support program that subsidizes corn and soybean production—crops, now predominantly GM, that result in serious soil erosion and water pollution from agrichemicals— at an estimated $ 12.2 billion. Such subsidies are a disincentive to farmers to adopt more ecologically sound farming practices.

This Life Science industry, rising from its agribusiness commodity-crop, pet food, petrochemical fertilizer and pharmaceutical roots, became a star of investor hope in the World Trade Organization's new world order, and with free trade blessings. But its promises of better seeds and crops through genetic engineering that will benefit all, in spite of a now almost global domination, has caused far more harm to many than any good. The indirect and unforeseen costs far outweigh the short term benefits, which more and more governments and businesses are beginning to realize.

The Life Science industry employs scientists to defend GM crops and the genetic engineering and cloning of farm animals, like oil companies employed scientists to say that global warming/climate change was a myth. They gave billions to Universities, setting up Chairs, Departments, Fellowships and lucrative consultative and patent sharing agreements, along with the US Chamber of Commerce.

Conclusions

From the above review it is evident that organic agriculture and holistic human and veterinary medicine have major roles to play in the end of days, as some call the collapse of the dominant culture of industrialism and consumerism, to help save our humanity from extinction, and the life and beauty of the natural world. They have major roles to play because they are of a different world view and bioethical basis than the dominant one of today that ignores the insight of Albert Einstein that the problems of the world cannot be solved at the same level of consciousness that caused them. This major role is not simply in better nutrition and health for all, but in the evolution of human species from a killer ape and global parasitic infestation to one that strives compassionately to establish a more symbiotic and co-creative relationship with the entire biotic community of this living Earth where peace, justice and respect for all life unify us in our sufferings and joy.

In the light of current trends, —from climate change and its catastrophic global socioeconomic, environmental, agricultural and public health consequences, to the devastation being caused by a foundering WTO in these times of escalating conflicts, failing economies, resources, and markets, and rising populations and epidemics of disease and violence—the bioethical imperative of humane, sustainable, socially just and organically certified agriculture is enlightened self-interest. It is the highest form of altruism if we care not only for our own health and that of the planet, but also for the rights and interests of indigenous peoples, endangered species like wolf and whale, elephant and albatross, and the last of the wild: And conserve and preserve our native seed stocks and animal breeding stock for that more enlightened future. As the Pennsylvania Dutch farmers say, "We do not inherit the land from our ancestors, we borrow it from our children."

There will be no tomorrows for today's good seed- savers unless the children of damnation awaken to Earth's sorrows and reverence all Creation.

Some sage once said, " Until we suffer the Earth and all living beings as we suffer for ourselves and for our own kind, there will be no end to suffering." And as the late Loren Eiseley observed, "We do not find ourselves until we see ourselves in the eyes of those who are other than human."

My friend Thomas Berry wrote 'The glory of the human has become the desolation of the earth. This I would consider an appropriate way to summarize the twentieth century.' But for me, I find seeds of hope in the practice and bioethics of humane, organic, and sustainable agriculture that can see us through the next century to a more enlightened and viable future.

Postscript: Ethics and Trade

A quasi-ethical framework can be fabricated on primarily economic criteria, under the banner of "sustainability." This is the situation with GATT (General Agreement on Trade and Tariffs) and the WTO (World Trade Organization), and much of the international accord that the 1992 United Nations' Conference on Environment and Development, the Rio Earth Summit, concocted. From the narrow materialistic perspective of GATT participants (who subsequently under pressure from public interest groups promised side-agreement correctives), a new world order for the human species was completed and ready to fly under the flag of world free trade.

The 'new world order' created globalization of industrialism, drawing countries rich and poor into a world market economy. This is a formula for disaster if there are no ethical constraints to protect the environment, biodiversity, wild and domestic animals, human rights (especially labor laws and consumer safety), and cultural diversity. The World Trade Organization, comprised of international business bureaucrats, is already a shadow world government that sees the world as a vast marketplace. As economist David Korten says in his book *When Corporations Rule the World*, most development interventions that use foreign aid financing "transfer control of local resources to ever larger and more centralized institutions that are unaccountable to the people and unresponsive to their needs."

This new world order, given the right ethical constraints, could become a formula for world peace and international cooperation, but only when the self-reliance of indigenous communities is coupled with sustainable local economies. It is unwise to create a dependence upon import-export markets because they are invariably volatile and can jeopardize national sovereignty and local economic security.

David Korten in his book *The Tyranny of the Global Economy* has shown why the public should not trust these powers but instead should reclaim their political power and reestablish localized economies. He summarizes his position as follows:

"The global economy has become like a malignant cancer, advancing the colonization of the planet's living spaces for the benefit of powerful corporations and financial institutions. It has turned these once useful institutions into instruments of a market tyranny that is destroying livelihoods, displacing people, and feeding on life in an insatiable quest for money. It forces us all to act in ways destructive of ourselves, our families, our communities, and nature. Human survival depends on a community-based, people-centered alternative beyond the failed extremist ideologies of communism and capitalism. This alternative is already being created through the initiatives of millions of people around the world who are taking back control of their lives and communities to create places where people can live and grow in balance with the living earth."

The globalization of bioethics through the WTO and GATT, in the face of looming socio-economically devastating climate change, is clearly a moral and a survival imperative. The core principles of sustainability and equitability as set out below are applicable also to other industries and philanthropic aid and development programs.

The Eight Bioethical Principles of Humane, Organic, Sustainable Agriculture

1. Humane sustainable organic agriculture (HOSA) entails the production of domestic animal protein and fiber on the economically prudent basis of an ecologically sound animal husbandry and the wise and appropriate use of natural resources. Such husbandry aims to enhance or at least protect the natural biodiversity of indigenous wild plant and animal species, and does not result in environmental degradation and pollution.
2. HOSA is socially just, respecting human rights and interests, especially those of indigenous peoples and native, peasant, and family-farm cultures and traditions, since the preservation of cultural diversity has inherent value just as does the preservation and enhancement of natural biodiversity.
3. HOSA recognizes the connections between farm worker health and safety, consumer health and farm animal health and well-being. It respects the right of consumers of animal protein to wholesome and healthful produce derived from animals whose basic physiological, behavioral, and social needs and requirements, which are integral to their overall health and well-being, are fully satisfied by the methods of husbandry that are practiced. The use of veterinary drugs to maintain animal health and productivity is minimized by the adoption of humane animal husbandry practices, which in turn lowers consumer health risks.

4. Furthermore, animals' health and overall well-being are maximized, rather than sacrificed to maximize productivity. Maximal, sustainable productivity is linked with optimal animal welfare, which in turn is linked with the optimal carrying capacity of the environment and availability of renewable natural resources.

5. HOSA is bioregionally appropriate, if not autonomous, linking livestock and poultry production with ecologically sound, organic crop and forage production systems and/or environmentally sound rangeland management.

6. HOSA does not engage in the import or export of any agricultural commodities, especially meat, wool, hides and animal feedstuffs, that have been produced at the expense of natural biodiversity and nonrenewable resources, and which undermine the rights and interests of local farmers and other indigenous people who practice sustainable, ecologically sound and socially just agriculture.

7. HOSA philosophically, is based upon the aphorism that we do not inherit the land, we borrow it from our children; it is ours only in sacred trust. This means, therefore, that HOSA entails respect and reverence for all life, its philosophy being Creation- or Earth-centered. It therefore embraces concern for the rights and interests of people, animals, and the environment. By so doing, it reconciles conflicting claims and concerns with the absolute right of all life to a whole and healthy environment and to equal and fair consideration.

8. HOSA provides the foundation for a community of hope and of a planetary democracy, whereby world peace, justice, and the integrity of Creation may be better assured. It leads to the recovery of culture, agriculture being the cultivation of the land and the production of food based on a hallowing covenant that commits us to the sacred obligation of caring for the Earth by farming with less harm and eating with conscience.

The "Blue Revolution" Seafood Industry

The 'Blue Revolution' programs to increase aquaculture/seafood production, purportedly to help feed the poor and to provide income for impoverished coastal communities, have caused much harm. So called farm-raised salmon in crowded floating cages are highly stressed, develop various diseases that mean pesticides and other drugs are prescribed that in turn wreak havoc on marine life and coastal ecosystems. The fish-by-catch meal fed to salmon is loaded with dioxins and PCBs, which concentrate in the salmon and pose a major consumer health risk equal to if not surpassing the mercury-load risk to consumers of tuna, sword fish and other top-of the marine food-chain predators. Commercial shrimp production has meant the destruction of mangrove and other wetlands, serious marine pollution, (like the commercial salmon industry), costly high-protein feed inputs, and many disease problems from intensive (and inhumane) aquatic animal husbandry and primitive veterinary care. This Blue Revolution, coupled with the vast drift-net factory fishing boats off shore, now means even greater poverty and malnutrition for once viable and self-sustaining indigenous fishing communities around the world. Those communities in the North, like the Alaskan Inuit Eskimos, are now at risk because of contaminated seafood that was their traditional diet and way of life as hunters of sea and ice. Mercury, PCBs, organochlorines and a host of dioxins now heavily contaminate halibut, seals, polar bears and whales, as well as the Eskimos, whose immune systems and general health are now seriously compromised. Their plight is not of their own making, now further compromised by the ice melting and the Arctic ecosystem collapsing all around them.

CHAPTER 10
Genetic Engineering & Cloning in Animal Agriculture: Bioethical & Food Safety Concerns

Synopsis: Farm Animal Cloning & Genetic Engineering
The farming of animals for human medical and other commercial/industrial purposes is being intensified through two new biotechnologies. One is genetic engineering that involves the splicing of alien genes into target animal embryos to create 'transgenic' animals, or the deletion of certain genes to create 'knockout' genetically modified animals. The other is cloning, that entails taking cells from the desired type of animal, that may be transgenic or a 'knockout', or from a conventionally bred genotype possessing such qualities as rapid growth or high milk or wool yield, and inserting the nuclei of these cells into the emptied ova from donor animals of the same species. Once activated by electrical fusion of the nucleus to the egg wall, these embryo-developing ova are inserted into surrogate mothers to be gestated.

Successful gene-splicing techniques and lines of transgenic and knockout animals, along with many varieties of transgenic crops, notably corn, cotton, rice, and soy bean, have been patented by the US government, university-biotechnology industry developers and investors, and most notably by the multinational pharmaceutical and 'life science' industries like Monsanto.

The pros and cons, costs and consequences of these forms of extreme biological manipulation for human profit will be examined in terms of who are the primary beneficiaries and losers from an objective, veterinary bioethical perspective.

Introduction: Pros & Cons
Advocates for the creation of genetically engineered and cloned animals claim that this new biotechnology is simply an extension of the process of human-directed natural selection for desired genetic traits that began thousands of years ago when animals were first domesticated. Some of these 'production' traits, coupled with how these animals are husbanded in crowded 'factory' farms, (see synopsis below) are now recognized as

causing a host of animal health, welfare, public health, and environmental problems.

Agricultural biotechnologists also contend that their patented transgenic or GM/GE (genetically modified/genetically engineered) crops are 'substantially equivalent' to conventional crops, and therefore are safe. Investors hope to profit also from the patents they hold on transgenic and cloned animals, just as they seek to monopolize the global market with their patented transgenic seeds.

Critics contend that the creation of transgenic and knockout animals, and cloning, are biologically aberrant (if not abhorrent) technologies that the life science industry and others cannot, from any sound scientific or bioethical basis, claim to be simply an extension of natural selective breeding. Clones are not identical to the original foundation-prototype because of epigenetic environmental influences and different maternal mitochondrial DNA. Likewise, GE crops are substantially different from conventional crops because the biotechnology employed for gene insertions and deletions is unnatural, and the consequences unpredictable by virtue of the inherent uncertainties of gene expression related to inaccurate and relatively crude gene-manipulations, and higher incidence of spontaneous mutations.

Animal Health & Welfare

Animal health and welfare advocates have documented the diseases and suffering that occur as a consequence of natural selective breeding to intensify animal productivity in terms of accelerated growth rates, greater body/flesh mass and higher milk production. Cloning such conventionally bred and genetically engineered animals, often raised under inhumane, intensive/confinement conditions, to create flocks and herds of more productive and profitable livestock, is now well under way in several countries. Commercial aims are directed toward developing animals that have leaner and more meat and healthful fats for human consumption (such as pigs that produce omega 3 fatty acids); greater disease resistance, fertility, and fecundity; produce more wool, milk with higher protein, even 'hypoallergenic' and analog human 'infant milk' high in human lactoferrin; and that produce environmentally less harmful wastes containing lower levels of phosphorus. Pigs with transgenes from spinach, jelly fish, and a marine worm, have been cloned. The spinach gene is employed to lower saturated fats and increase linoleic acid levels in body fat; the jellyfish gene to make the pigs fluorescent, thus serving as a genetic marker; and the nematode worm gene to convert omega 6 fatty acids into more consumer-beneficial omega 3 fatty acids. In the US, goats may become the future 'bioreactors', producing proteins in their mammary glands for use in human medicine. Both foundation animals and F1 generation transgenic pigs with spinach desaturase gene (inserted to convert saturated fats into unsaturated linoleic acid) had high mortality rates. Cloned transgenic cattle have been produced that have human monoclonal antibodies in their blood, like human immunoglobulin and melanoma attacking antibodies. There are great market hopes in this field of animal pharming.

The FDA (U.S. Food & Drug Administration) in 2008 announced that the meat and milk from cloned cattle, pigs, is as safe to eat as food from more conventionally bred animals. But concerns over people eating meat and dairy products from cloned animals have nothing to do with any foreseeable risk to consumers. The inherent danger of genetic uniformity in cloned herds selected for production traits that are already linked with various production-related health and welfare problems is a serious ethical issue. Greater genetic uniformity can mean significant economic losses from diseases that become contagious when there is a fatal combination of genetic susceptibility and uniformity. The propagation, by accident or design, of unhealthy traits in cloned and genetically engineered breeds which would result in disease, miscarriages, birth defects etc, have been well documented in the scientific literature. The loss of genetic diversity in the livestock population increasingly displaced and replaced by homozygous clones is a bioethical and potential financial issue that governments and regulatory agencies have not fully addressed.

The treatment and ultimate fate of surrogate and donor cattle and other farmed animals used as mere instruments of biotechnology call for the most rigorous humane standards and their effective enforcement by the US and other governments.

Some of the first farmed animals in nonpharmaceutical production to be cloned have been high-yielding dairy cows. Since animal bioengineers from the US and Japan have collaboratively succeeded in genetically engineered cattle to be resistant to BSE—bovine spongioform encephalopathy, or mad cow disease—animals like theirs may well be the first to be vigorously propagated through artificial insemination and cloning technology. Regardless, BSE was essentially a human-created disease following the livestock industry practice of recycling dead animals back into the food chain in livestock feed. (This epidemic that devastated the UK's cattle industry may have originated, according to some epidemiologists, from contaminated cattle remains imported from India for incorporation into livestock feed.)

Transgenic farm animals are already being cloned to create flocks and herds for 'gene pharming', many carrying human genes that make them produce various novel proteins in their milk, like antithrombin 111 and alpha-trypsin that the pharmaceutical industry seeks to profit by. The animals are called mammary bioreactors. The global market for such recombinant proteins from domestic animals is expected to reach US&18.6 billion by 2013, but similar proteins from transgenic pharm crops producing pharmacologically active proteins may lower this figure considerably.

In the spring of 2009 the US government (FDA) approved GTC Biotherapeutics' transgenic (GE) goat anti-coagulant biopharmaceutical for commercial production from a herd of 200 GE goats, without giving any call for public comment. PharmAthene of Annapolis Maryland is reportedly developing a treatment for nerve gas poisoning from the milk of GE goats.

Genetically altered farm animals are also being created to serve as organ donors for humans; to produce human blood substitutes, and to produce monoclonal and polyclonal antibodies. The presence of retroviruses in pig livers and other organs make the risks of xenotransplantation considerable, some virologists calling for a prohibition on putting immuno-humanized pig organs into human patients. Models of human diseases have also been created in transgenic animals, like Denmark's cloned pigs that have genes for Alzheimer's disease, and pigs in the US being genetically engineered to serve as models for cystic fibrosis in humans. According to a 2005 public survey by the Pew Initiative on Food and biotechnology, 56 percent of Americans oppose research into genetic modification of animals.

Veterinary, Ecological & Biological Issues

The incorporation of other species' genes into farm animals, like the human growth hormone gene into pigs, can have so called multiple deleterious pleiotropic effects. These unforeseen consequences on transgenic animals' development and physiology include abnormal and excessive bone growth (acromegaly), arthritis, skin and eye problems, peptic ulcers, pneumonia, pericarditis and diarrhea (implying impaired immune systems), as well as decreased male libido and disruption of estrus cycles. Inserted/spliced genes may be 'overxpressed', meaning overactive, and produce excessive amounts of certain proteins like growth hormone, or create an 'insertional mutation' problem, disrupting the functions of other genes and organ systems.

These Russian roulette-like adverse consequences of genetic engineering can result in serious health problems later in life if they do not cause fetal deformities and pre- or early postnatal death. Many transgenic creations are either still-born or are resorbed by the mother; or soon after birth they die from internal organ failure or circulatory, or immune system collapse. This is especially so with cloned animals, the success rate being extremely low in terms of survivability. For example, a US Dept of Agriculture research experiment to create cows resistant to mastitis had a success rate of 1.5 percent, 8 calves being born from 330 transgenic cloned ova, only eight of these being gestated to term as live calves. Three of these died before maturity.

Cloning can result in abnormally large fetuses that can mean suffering and death for the mothers. Abnormal placentas deformed still-born fetuses, and live offspring with defective lungs, hearts, brains, kidneys, immune systems, and suffering from circulatory problems, deformed faces, feet and tendons, intestinal blockages and diabetes have been documented. Cloning seems more likely to cause problems when the cloned animals have been previously subjected to genetic engineering. Yet it is only through cloning that productive flocks and herds can be quickly built from one or two 'founder' transgenic/knockout stock.

Unacceptable Animal Biotechnology
The incorporation of cloned and transgenic farm animals into conventional, industrial agriculture is ethically, economically and environmentally unacceptable. This is because it is being directed primarily toward making confinement-raised farmed animals (and aquatic species on fish farms, notably transgenic salmon) more 'productive'. This is a myth because the industrialized factory farming of animals is not only inhumane and environmentally damaging; it is also not sustainable economically or ecologically. It is blight across most rural landscapes throughout much of the industrial world, and, according to a recent report by the United Nation's FAO, (Food and Agriculture Organization), it is a major culprit in global warming, when coupled with the enormous global population of livestock that are creating desert wastelands from over-stocking and over-grazing in less developed countries.

Health and environmental experts, conservationists and economists are calling for a reduction in livestock numbers globally, and for more sustainable, organic and ecological farming practices, including more humane and 'free range' animal production methods. They see no place for cloned livestock and agricultural bioengineering if there is to be a viable future for sustainable agriculture.

The Western market and unhealthy appetite for animal products as a dietary staple, that the inhumane farm animal industry promotes through government subsidies and price supports at tax payer's expense, is now being exported to many developing countries, most notably by the World Bank, at great cost to their natural biodiversity, traditional, sustainable farming practices, and to environmental and public health. We should all ask what farm animal cloning and genetic engineering have to do with feeding the poor and hungry, and in developing a sustainable and socially just agriculture locally and globally, to feed the starving millions of our kind, without further sacrifice of biodiversity, the Earth's wild plant and animal species, and most precious communities, notably those recognized by the UN as Global Biosphere Reserves.

All countries importing genetically engineered seeds, and foods and animal feeds derived there from, as well as meat and dairy products from cloned animals, should, for the above bioethical, scientifically verifiable, environmental, and economic reasons, immediately boycott this market sector of agricultural and animal production biotechnology: And cease and desist from further endeavors to develop their own animal and plant biotechnologies that are no substitute for humane, sustainable, socially just, ecologically sound and environmentally beneficial food and fiber production methods.

Exploiting farm animals as medical models of human diseases, and as sources of new pharmaceutical and other medical products, from livers to hearts for 'xenotransplantation' into humans, raises a host of public health and bioethical questions. It may not be a sustainable or effective path for medicine to take, profitability notwithstanding. From a bioethical perspective it puts the human in the role of genetic parasite, which, from a cultural and evolutionary perspective, may not make for a better or desirable future.

Cloned, transgenic farm animals created for human consumption are likely to be kept under the same pathogenic husbandry conditions and subjected to the same kinds of inhumane treatment to which conventionally bred livestock and poultry are currently subjected. The reasons include custom, convenience, economies of scale, and prioritizing profit margins over animal health and welfare. Those created to serve as organ-donors and to supply various biologics or pharmaceutical products will be cared for in proportion to their invested value and productive worth.

The cavalier attitude toward the widespread use of vaccines to control farmed animal and human diseases, most of which are modified/ attenuated live, or genetically modified live strains, is of epidemiological concern. Diseases in nontarget species have been documented, and the possibilities of new viral strains evolving through recombination opens a Pandora's Box that is the antithesis of preventive medicine, vaccinations being sold under that erroneous banner.

We all need to ask what kind of world we are creating through industrial, biomedical and agricultural biotechnology, splicing and silencing genes, manipulating viruses, inserting artificial chromosomes, and creating clones. To the instrumental rationalist, minimizing, (and even discounting) human health and environmental risks, and avoiding animal suffering whenever possible, are the sole ethical criteria for acceptability Are these new biotechnologies really part of some enlightened vision of a sustainable future, or are they paving the way to an ever more depraved and desperate existence for the next generation?

Future Directions: Bioethical Choices

The avaricious quickening of industrialism and consumerism has created a non sustainable and unethical enterprise system that can only be made to cause less harm by all of we Earth consumers voting with our dollars. We should eschew all manufactured, processed and prepared (pre-pared) foods, and ideally prepare our own meals from organically certified whole foods, or purchase prepared foods that are organic and whole rather than highly processed. This same initiative should be applied to what companion animals are given to eat, for their own health, and indirectly for the health of the environment by supporting more sustainable, and humane farming and food-production methods.

All consumers need to take a stand and use their purchasing power to support humane, sustainable organic food producers and retailers for the good of the environment, farm animals, farmers who care, and for their own health and that of their animal companions. Just as more and more doctors and other human health care professionals are advocating healthier diets and a healthier agriculture, so should all veterinarians and those organizations and individuals concerned about the health and welfare of both companion and farm animals.

CHAPTER 11
Genetic Chaos?
Genetically Engineered Ingredients in Pet Foods, Livestock
Feed & Human Foods & Beverages: Consumer beware!

The inclusion of genetically engineered crops and feed additives in
livestock and poultry feed, in pet foods, and directly into the human food
chain, especially in processed foods and beverages containing corn and soy
ingredients, is a major health concern for reasons that I will document.

Genetically engineered (GE)/genetically modified (GM) plants –
"Frankenfoods" to critics- contain artificially inserted genes from viruses,
bacteria, other plant species, also from insects, humans, and other animals.
This process can result in entirely novel chemicals being produced that
were never in our foods or what farmed and companion animals were ever
fed before. Also normal nutrients may become deficient as a consequence
of alien gene insertion, while other naturally occurring plant substances
may become so concentrated as to become toxic.

GE plants are created primarily to increase their resistance to
herbicides and insect pests. Both the US government and the multinational
corporations patenting and selling these seeds of potential destruction
to farmers to plant crops that go to human, pet food and livestock feed
manufacturers would have us believe that GE crops and food ingredients
are safe, and that to believe otherwise is to not trust in science and progress.

In 2006, an estimated 136 million acres of U.S. cropland was
used to grow GM crops. Some 89% of soybeans and 61% of corn crops
are now genetically engineered. Canola is also genetically engineered,
and vegetable oils (canola and corn) along with soy protein and lecithin,
are used widely in a variety of prepared foods for people and their pets.
Genetically engineered sugar beet will soon be planted widely as a source
of sugar for the food industry. Beet pulp is a common ingredient in pet
foods. GM wheat is also on the horizon.

Commodity producers' adoption of GE crops in the US,
prohibited in many other countries, has been dramatic, according the US
Dept. of Agriculture (See their Graph below).

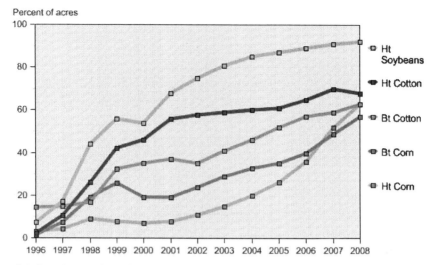

Percent of acres

Data for each crop category include varieties with both HT and Bt (stacked) traits.
Source: 1996-1999 data are from Fernandez-Cornejo and McBride (2002).

Figure 11-1. Rapid Growth of Genetically Engineered Crops in the US (Based on USDA/ERS)

This adoption by contracted producers is not unexpected since a handful of powerful pharmaceutical and agrichemical multinational corporations like Bayer and Monsanto, have gained a monopolistic control over the major commodity crop seed stocks, making available to farmers only their highly promoted, patented varieties of GE seeds. Farmers then sell these commodities to livestock feed companies and to the food, beverage, candy and cosmetic industries like Mars Inc., Nestle`, Colgate-Palmolive Co., and Procter and Gamble Inc. These four multinationals monopolize the pet food industry selling such familiar and widely advertised brands as Hill's Science Diet, Purina, Pedigree, Iams, and Eukanuba. It is no coincidence that Pet Health Insurance schemes are being marketed by one of these companies.

In essence the main-stream pet food industry, a subsidiary of agribusiness, profitably recycles human food and beverage industry by-products, and livestock and poultry parts considered unfit for human consumption, into pet foods. (For details see *Not Fit for a Dog: The Truth About Manufactured Dog and Cat Food*, ref. below)

"Stacked" gene varieties are those containing GE traits for both herbicide tolerance (HT) and insect resistance (Bt).

Some of the Risks

Numerous issues and unanswered questions surround the "safety" of these GE/GM crops and foods. In their recent review, Dona & Arvanitoyannis (2009) conclude that 'The results of most of the rather few studies conducted with GM foods indicate that they may cause hepatic, pancreatic, renal, and reproductive effects and may alter hematological, biochemical, and immunologic parameters the significance of which remains unknown. The above results indicate that many GM foods have some common toxic effects. Therefore, further studies should be conducted in order to elucidate the mechanism dominating this action. Small amounts of ingested DNA may not be broken down under digestive processes and there is a possibility that this DNA may either enter the bloodstream or be excreted, especially in individuals with abnormal digestion as a result of chronic gastrointestinal disease or with immunodeficiency'.

The insecticidal poison Bt (*Bacillus thuringiensis*) is present in most genetically engineered U.S. commodity crops that go into animal feed and pet foods. High levels of Bt toxin in GM crops have made farmers ill and poisoned farm animals eating crop residues. Bt toxin harms microorganisms in the soil vital to plant health, high levels being created when GM crop residues are mulched or ploughed into the soil.

- Genetic material in GM herbicide resistant soybeans can be transferred to bacteria in our digestive systems. This means that foreign proteins could be manufactured in our own digestive systems by such bacteria, turning them into pesticide factories.
- So called "overexpression" can occur when spliced genes that manufacture chemicals such as Bt become hyperactive inside the plant and result in potentially toxic plant tissues. These are lethal not just to meal worms and other crop pests, but also to, birds, butterflies, other wildlife, and possibly to humans and their pets.
- The herbicides glufosinate and glyphosate are liberally applied across the U.S. and in many other countries to millions of acres of crops genetically engineered to be resistant to these herbicides. These poisons are actually absorbed by the crops, while all else growing in the fields and much of the surrounding aquatic life in rivers and lakes, and are wiped out. These widely used herbicides and the additives therein have caused kidney damage and other health problems in animals; can cause endocrine disruption, trigger birth defects in frogs and are lethal to many aquatic species. Glyphosate has been linked with non-Hodgkin lymphoma, miscarriages and premature births in humans.

- These herbicides and other agrichemicals, along with the insecticide Bt, are found in pet foods and the crops and crop by-products fed to cattle, pigs, poultry, and dairy cows.

Many nutritionists and other health experts are linking the rise in human food allergies—skin problems and inflammatory/irritable bowel syndromes— to the increased consumption of GM foods and food additives, especially genetically engineered soy products that contain novel proteins.

- Almost every independent animal feeding safety study has shown adverse or unexplained effects of GM foods, including: Inflammation and abnormal cell growth (possibly pre-cancerous) in the stomach and small intestines; abnormal development, inflammation, and cellular changes in the liver, kidney, testicles, heart, pancreas, brain; and poor growth and higher mortalities than normal.

Three crucial papers, one demonstrating reduced fertility in mice fed on a diet including NK603xMON810 maize; another demonstrating damage to the immune system in mice fed on a diet including MON810 maize; and yet another showing significant histopathological changes in liver and kidney in rats fed with BT maize (probably MON810) have been recently published. (See references below).

- Researchers have found that unlike conventionally bred crops, GM varieties are intrinsically unstable and prone to spontaneous mutations. When mutations occur, you can never know if what is being grown, harvested, processed and consumed is really safe and nutritious.
- The inserted genes can have unforeseen consequences, so called multiple pleiotropic effects. These unpredictable consequences of introducing a new genetic trait or quality include alterations in existing gene function and relationships with other genes. A dramatic example of this in animals is in the genetically engineered pigs that were created to carry human growth genes at the U.S. government's research facility in Beltsville Maryland. These pigs became cripples, suffering from multiple health problems including arthritis, bone-growth deformities, and had impaired immune and reproductive systems. Multiple pleiotropic effects in GM soy include excesses of certain phytoestrogens, and the presence of anti-nutrient substances, some of which could be a consequence of genomic interaction with

mutagenic agrichemicals compounded by the poor nutrition (and nutritive value) of conventionally, rather than organically grown crops.

- GM seeds are genetically unstable because they are more prone than normal to undergo spontaneous mutations. This can mean that GM crops could produce novel, harmful proteins, excessive, even toxic amounts of normal nutrients, or become extremely deficient in same: Spontaneous mutations = genetic roulette.
- The delicate bacterial balance in the digestive systems of man and beast alike is disrupted by herbicide food residues and possibly by the mutagenic, unknown consequences of transgenic DNA segments (from the genes of all GM foods) becoming incorporated into the bacterial DNA.
- The widely employed Cauliflower mosaic virus (CaMV) used as a vector for transgenes in plants has an insertional/recombination 'hot spot' that is prone to break and recombine with other DNA and plant mRNA and RNA viruses. Novel viruses containing transgenes, and bacteria with antibiotic marker transgenes may then develop with potentially devastating consequences to natural and agricultural ecosystems. Some virologists note CaMV is related to and could recombine with Hepatitis B and HIV viruses. Infected people consuming large numbers of virus genes in GM crops could become incubators for new virus strains created through recombination with CaMV.

My advice to consumers and pet owners alike is to look for the USDA Organic certification label on foods since the government has resisted attempts to have GE/GM products appropriately labeled. Read the labels on prepared foods and avoid those that contain corn and soy products, (including cooking oils) since these are most likely to have come from GE/GM crops. Corn and soy ingredients have no place in pet foods, especially in cat foods, even if they are from conventional, non-GE/GM varieties, because of their association with a variety of health problems in companion animals. These include allergies, skin problems, periodontal disease, inflammatory bowel disease, and cystitis. (For details see www. twobitdog.com/drfox/). But they are widely used because of their low cost as cheap sources of calories and protein.

Doctors Warn: Avoid Genetically Modified Food

The American Academy of Environmental Medicine states, "Genetically Modified foods have not been properly tested and pose a serious health risk. There is more than a casual association between GM foods and adverse health effects. There is causation."

For more details go tohttp://www.sentienttimes.com/09/June_July_09/doctors.html

One of the first government employed scientist to blow the whistle on the health risks and unproven safety of GM foods was immediately fired. He worked for the same British government laboratory that collaborated with China to develop genetically engineered wheat. This good scientist, Dr. Arapad Pusztai, whose research findings he has now shared with millions of concerned consumers around the world, were suppressed and loudly discredited by the Life Science government-industry-university complex. Their act of suppression gave Dr. Pusztai his world forum, and he came to this as an objective scientist with no bias pro or con GM foods. (For considerable documentation, see references below).

The agricultural biotechnology industry that calls itself the 'life science industry' with its patented varieties of genetically engineered/GM/gene-modified/transgenic seeds grew out of the vested interests of the petrochemical-pharmaceutical-agribusiness complex in monopolizing world agriculture. It succeeded, in spite of public outcry, in gaining government approval to market GM seeds at home and abroad, insisting, without any documented scientific evidence, that its patented seeds were safe, and so there would be no risks to consumers or of significant harm to the environment.

I believe that this is the most egregious, if not heinous business activity of the 21st century, and that there is now sufficient scientific evidence for a class action suit against all multinational corporations and allied governments to not only compensate farmers whose seed stocks and crops have been genetically contaminated by pollen drift from GM crops, but to also pay for a total recall of all such crops and seeds that are so prevalent as to now contaminate most basic food commodities. Ecosystems will have to be monitored for years, and all harvests, until the aberrant genetic constructs and toxic and mutagenic properties of GM crop origin are removed from the germ- lines of domesticated plants and their wild relatives.

The US government even attempted to have genetically engineered seeds and foods included under the National Organic Standards, but were blocked by public outcry and a deluge of close to

300,000 letters of protest. Genetically engineered crops of corn, soy and canola that are herbicide resistant, and corn that produces its own insecticidal poison called Bt, get into the human food chain, and are put into livestock feed and pet foods with the government's blessing: And quite probably to the demise of the honey bee and a large agricultural sector of bee-pollination dependent orchard and field crops.

In the 2007 US Farm Bill, the government will be distributing some $33 billion in subsidies to 'help' the nations' farmers over the next 5 years. But in actuality around 65 percent of these tax dollars will go to 10 percent of the recipients. These are the big producers of these increasingly genetically engineered 'commodity crops' that go into processed foods as soy protein, corn gluten and syrup, wheat flour and bran, rice flour, and oils of soy, corn and canola, with cotton byproducts being put into livestock feed, and more corn going in to the speculative and short-sighted bio-fuels market. Genetically engineered sugar beet will soon be planted widely as a source of sugar for the food industry. Only wheat, of these commodity crops, is not genetically engineered.

That only 2 percent of this agricultural spending will go to support vegetable and other whole food producers confirms the insanity in these times of corporate and investor cupidity and consumer stupidity and gullibility.

In 2006, an estimated 136 million acres of U.S. cropland was used to grow GM crops -89% of soybeans, 83% of cotton, and 61% of corn crops were genetically engineered. Canola is also genetically engineered, and vegetable oils (cotton, canola and corn) along with soy protein and lecithin, are used widely in a variety of prepared foods for people and their pets. Genetically engineered sugar beet will soon be planted widely as a source of sugar for the food industry. Beet pulp is a common ingredient in pet foods.

Since the FDA does not insist on the labeling of human or pet foods when they contain GM ingredients, we have no way of knowing what we are really eating or feeding to our pets: Unless, that is, there is the green USDA label saying USDA ORGANIC, indicating Organic Certification. Many manufacturers may also label their product GM FREE or NO GM INGREDIENTS.

The compiled references at the end of this book on the health and environmental hazards of genetically engineered crops and foods provide sufficient scientific support for such correctives and initiatives that are indeed in most urgent need of being implemented if the natural biodiversity and vitality of the plants and plant-based ecosystems of the world are to be protected and restored. It is already evident that new disease complexes can be triggered by GM foods in animals and humans that are extremely challenging to diagnose and treat. The best and only preventive is Organically Certified food.

Perhaps in some more enlightened age, activities like those of the agri-biotechnology industry and the entire FDA complex, would be outlawed and prosecuted as Crimes against Nature as well as against Humanity.

CHAPTER 12
The Bioethics & Politics of Manufactured Pet Foods

Synopsis
Where, how, and what kinds of crops are grown; where and how livestock
and poultry are raised and treated; and how the foods derived there
from are processed that we and our animal companions eventually
consume, have profound consequences that call for bioethical evaluation
and accountability. The hidden costs of the dominant, multinational,
agribusiness food production system, of which the pet food industry is a
highly profitable and politically influential subsidiary, concern and involve
us all as consumers; and in particular as veterinarians, because of the
animal health, welfare, economic, and ecological implications of clients
feeding conventional manufactured pet foods to their dogs and cats.
Examined from this broader bioethical perspective, what people select to
feed their pets and consume for themselves in the future must be based
upon sound science, ethics, and informed choice. Both the government
and the FDA—the Food-Drug-Agribusiness industrial complex— must
held accountable and be responsive to public demand and right to
guaranteed food quality and safety standards (regardless of country of
origin), and for foods derived from humane, sustainable, socially just, and
organically certified farming systems.

Bioethical Questions
There are several ethical areas of concern that need to be considered in
determining the kind and quality of food that people should give to their
animal companions. The term bioethics rather than ethics is preferable
because ethics has more to do with how we behave toward each other,
while bioethics has a broader scope. One definition of bioethics in my
book *Eating With Conscience: The Bioethics of Food,* is "the extension of ethical
issues and concerns from the immediate human community into the
broader biological dimension of our relations with and duties toward the
biotic community—animals, plants, and the whole of nature. Bioethical
principles in food production and consumption are the keys to a more
sensible and compassionate future."

The first area concerns the animals' welfare and respect for their basic rights. One of the basic rights or entitlements is the right, under our dominion, to a wholesome and healthful diet. It is a responsibility that all pet owners should willingly accept, and see as a moral duty to their animals since the animals have no choice but to eat whatever they are given.

Another area concerns the veterinary profession whose duty it is to advise their clients fully on all matters that may harm or enhance their client-animal's health. From a veterinary preventive and holistic medical perspective, right (optimal) nutrition is one of the four pillars of good practice and animal well-being (From a Paper presented at the American Holistic Veterinary medical Association 2008 Reno Conference).

Providing animals under our care with right nutrition, proper understanding, an optimal social environment, and freedom from inherited diseases are bioethical principles that need to be more widely understood and adopted by all the people, professions, industries, and institutions that have anything to do with animals, as well as profit from them.

Bioethics & Respect for Life

In addition to the bioethical imperative of putting compassionate concern and respect for all animals into action, there are other broad bioethical principles that are relevant to how we choose to live, feed ourselves and our pets, and impact the natural environment. We have a long way to go. A first step is to apply bioethics to agriculture and consumer food choices. In linking our own food choices with a more humane, sustainable and organic agriculture, we must also include our animal companions under the ethic of "eating with conscience." It is ethically inconsistent, costs notwithstanding, for us to claim to love and respect our companion animals and not have the same concern about the origins and quality of the food we give to them as we have for ourselves and for other human members of the family. We all need to care enough about farm animals, their suffering in agribusiness factory farms and feedlots, and the harmful environmental, wildlife, and public health problems caused by these industrialized livestock production systems, to help put an end to them. There will be no end in sight until we all eat and feed our pets with conscience.

The 'Science' of Pet Foods

The science of animal nutrition first evolved as an adjunct to farm animal husbandry, its primary emphasis being on maximizing profits through formulating livestock and poultry feeds that produce the best growth/ovulation/lactation at the least cost. Applying this kind of animal production science to the formulation of pet foods, a step-up for many companion animals that were hitherto often severely malnourished, and who suffered such nutritional deficiency diseases as rickets, and canine pellagra or black tongue, has been highly profitable. But based on the same animal production paradigm, a host of companion animal health problems have been created by most manufactured pet foods. Some of these parallel the so called 'metabolic syndrome', obesity-diabetes epidemic in the human population

Now veterinary clinical nutrition, coupled with nutritional genomics, are being called upon to help various pure bred, mutant varieties of dogs and cats avoid certain dietary ingredients that can make them ill, and to be prescribed special supplements to avert various nutrition-related diseases. Clinical nutrition for elderly humans is as deficient as it is for geriatric companion animals, the veterinary profession being more advanced, from my perspective, than the medical profession in this regard. Both professions parallel each other in addressing the special nutritional needs of patients with various chronic degenerative diseases like arthritis, cancer, heart and kidney disease. More are now recognizing that the best prevention is to not make manufactured, convenience foods for both people and pets their dietary staple. Many health problems are in part due to the nutritional flaws of manufactured, highly processed foods and whole-food byproducts, compounded by genomic variables. Epigenetic variables (influence of mother's diet on offspring) are also being recognized, and from a bioethical perspective, they underscore the precautionary principle. This principle should have been applied before pet food manufacturers decided to proclaim that their products were scientifically formulated, and therefore safe, 'complete and balanced', to provide for all of a pet's dietary needs. Nutritional genomics alone, rules this out such a statement as pure marketeerism without any scientific basis.

Nutritional epigenetics, for example, is revealing that mothers on a junk food diet have offspring who are highly susceptible to the same health problems as their mothers, like diabetes and obesity, and who actually prefer junk food over a more healthful diet. The nutritional status of the mother, and of the offspring during their formative postnatal period, can influence their cognitive and emotional development, disease resistance, fertility, fecundity, quality of life, and longevity. So we should regard the transgenerational consequences of manufactured pet foods on the health of companion animals as a major issue of holistic and preventive veterinary medicine, and a responsibility of breeders of dogs and cats to address. Dramatic evidence that diet affects offspring comes from the studies of Sonia de Assis et al, Georgetown University Medical Center, which showed that the offspring of rats whose mother's were fed a high fat diet were more prone to breast cancer. Most startling was the finding that even the offspring of daughters of rats fed a high fat diet, but who themselves were fed a normal diet, had a higher risk than normal of developing breast cancer when exposed to a carcinogen (*New Scientist*, April 20, 2010, report by Ewen Callaway). Rats on junk food pass cancer down generations.

The kinds of nutritional diseases attributable in part to highly processed pet foods mirror those seen especially amongst impoverished indigenous peoples who have been disenfranchised from their lands and from traditional, sustainable farming, fishing, and gathering and hunting economies and healthful diets to which, over generations, they have become biologically adapted. These people in particular are not biologically adapted to the kinds of food available in poorer communities, just as cats and dogs are not biologically adapted to manufactured, nutrient-deficient and imbalanced (too high cereal content) pet foods. The sudden generational switch to essentially unnatural diets, coupled with multiple negative environmental, social, and economic stressors, exposed genetic susceptibilities to a host of diseases, making some epidemic, like diabetes Type 2 with all its complications from blindness to amputations and life in a wheel chair for Arizona's Pima Indians and other impoverished indigenous peoples... High blood pressure, stroke, heart attacks, obesity, arthritis, gall bladder and liver disease, arteriosclerosis, various types of cancer, allergies, and other immune system disorders linked to elevated cortisol levels and associated development of arteriosclerosis and increased susceptibility to infections, depression, hopelessness/helplessness, alcoholism, drug addiction, pharmaceutical dependence, crime and violence are epidemic afflictions of impoverished and disenfranchised communities around the world. They are notably evident in the poorer communities of the more affluent developed industrial technocracies, where the Western diet and the appetites of mammon are the cause of much dis-ease (Mammon is where material riches are regarded as an object of worship and greedy pursuit). The annual costs of diabetes Type 2 in the US alone is around $20 billion.

The byproducts of this diet are fed back to livestock and poultry, and are the main ingredients of manufactured pet foods to which few pets are biologically adapted. Wild foods, from meats and herbs to fruits and vegetables, had higher nutrient content and far fewer harmful contaminants than any ingredient in the modern, so called Western diet, and no adulterants, synthetic additives or preservatives. Now for purported public health reasons, (but really because the food industry is dysfunctional and nonsustainable—unsafe at any cost), the FDA is proposing that meat and other perishable consumables should be irradiated: Foods not of the gods but of the disgodded.

Corporate Ethics & Politics

Veterinarian Dr. Lon D. Lewis, one of the first Diplomats of the American College of Veterinary Nutrition, sent me a personal communication on December 11, 1997, in which he stated:

"Commercial dog foods do not provide optimum nutrition, safety, or, to paraphrase your book title Eating with Conscience: The Bioethics of Food, to feed with a conscience—From 30 years in veterinary medicine and nutrition practice, teaching, consulting, research and development in private practice, academia and industry, I believe most pet food companies are doing a good job of providing nutrition for the amount that the foods cost, but not in providing optimum nutrition, food safety, and certainly not in promoting good agricultural, environmental and animal husbandry practices. Of course major human foods producing companies, as well as our government, I do not believe are doing much to promote the latter either…"

Let's revisit Dr. Lewis' statement that most pet food manufacturers are doing a good job of providing nutrition 'for the amount that the foods cost'. This is the crux of the problem with most manufactured pet foods— the economics of lowest-cost ingredients to satisfy minimal 'science-based' nutritional content in order to maximize, not quality but profit margins. As one Chinese businessman told the press, the pet food poisoning debacle of 2007 from wheat flour imported from China spiked with melamine and cyanuric acid that caused acute renal failure and killed thousands of cats and dogs, should have been suspect by the importers because it was too cheap to be sold as wheat gluten and rice protein.

What of corporate ethics in a business world where the bottom line is the profit margin and where consumer demand, based on trust, is manipulated through advertising propaganda and disinformation? These have become the 'collegiate' norms of market-driven policies and programs in a highly competitive global market economy. Until competition is eliminated via corporate mergers and monopolistic cartels, a competitive down-spiral in the quality of manufactured foods, including pet foods, is a market-driven reality. This down-spiral is created by a profit-margin factor determined by the ratio between ingredient, processing, marketing/advertising costs, and the wholesale price of the product.

Such productionism, as philosopher and agricultural ethicist Paul Thompson calls this market-driven process, is the dominant ethos of industrial society, and of agribusiness in particular, of which the pet food industry is a subsidiary and beneficiary, converting essentially condemned, and discarded food and beverage industry byproducts into a profitable product, companion animals being used as waste- recycling agents.

The silencing of corporate, government and nongovernment organization whistleblowers, the control of the media, and the enactment of laws like the Food Disparagement Act, serve to disenfranchise consumers from the realm of truth and from their right to know. Criminalizing free speech and unbiased professional opinion when vested interests and the status quo are perceived to be threatened, is a sign of how corrupt and surreal these Orwellian times have become.

British Broadcasting Corporation television canceled a scheduled interview in England with me where I was going to discuss my new book *Agricide: The Hidden Farm and Food Crisis that Affects Us All,* because the pet food, livestock and agribusiness industrial complex felt it was too threatening to have the harmful consequences of excessive livestock production and meat consumption exposed to the public after a documentary on world hunger contrasted the plight of the poor with how well pets are fed in Europe.

An increasingly monopolistic control over how our food is grown, processed, and marketed is a fact of the times that has implications in terms of consumer choice and right to know, and in terms of our health and the health of our animal companions. As consumers and public citizens we must all take a stand, and by voting with our dollars support those good farmers and food retailers who know that, as Chef Alice Waters observes, "Good food starts in fields and orchards well tended. This is knowledge that we ignore at our peril, for without good farming there can be no good food; and without good food there can be no good life."

Myth & Reality

The sheer convenience of opening a container of relatively low cost food for our dogs and cats, and the pet-food industry promotion of the many benefits of companion animals have combined to create a highly profitable (around $ 15 billion per year) branch of agribusiness. It has relied for too long on recycling cheap food industry byproducts unfit for human consumption; and on a very limited knowledge base and scientific evaluation of the nutritional adequacies and health risks of such ingredients, and of the various supplements and additives used to make pet foods not go bad or look bad, and conform to the National Research Council's minimum nutritional standards.

Some erroneous information has been spread by the pet food industry to the public and to veterinary students whose short course in animal nutrition was, until recently, usually taught by industry employees. One is that pets don't need variety and that switching brands and giving different kinds of food will cause digestive problems, or turns them into finicky eaters. Other myths that have no scientific or clinical credibility are that human food is bad for pets, and that an all-dry kibble diet is fine for cats because it keeps their teeth clean. Yet another myth is that because most commercial pet foods are scientifically formulated and balanced, feeding nutritious supplements is not necessary and even harmful because the "balance" of the diet may be upset. These unqualified generalizations are neither scientifically valid nor professionally ethical. Nor are the claims and even content information on pet food labels that follow a standardized format orchestrated by the nonregulatory American Association of Feed Control Officials. Claims such as 'providing complete nutrition' year after year have proven false a decade or so later when all the cases of pets who became sick were recognized by veterinarians as falling into a category where an essential nutrient has been found to be lacking, or a supplement put in at concentrations that turned out to be poisonous. As for FDA and USDA oversight of the pet food sector of agribusiness, the public hearings held following the largest pet food recall ever in 2007 revealed a wholly inadequate pet food quality and safety system, with no government regulatory power: and a human food-safety system, especially with regard for imported foods, supplements, and pharmaceuticals, to be in total disarray, under-funded, under-staffed, and essentially dysfunctional.

Note

The rumors about the unhealthy aspects of cow's milk, even when pasteurized, contributing to Type 1 diabetes, heart disease, even autism and schizophrenia, have been confirmed as being attributable to a certain type of cow's milk high in a beta-casein that forms when humans digest this milk. This milk is designated Type A1, and is a genetic mutation in cattle of European origin whose Type A2 milk does not contain this harmful protein. This mutant gene producing A1 milk has become endemic in herds n the U.S., Canada, New Zealand, Australia and northern Europe according to dairy researcher Keith Woodford. (See his book *Devil in the Milk: Illness, Health, and the Politics of A1 and A2 Milk*. Boston: Chelsea Green Pubs, 2009).

Postscript: Natural & Unnatural History of Pet Food & Feeding
There are several aspects of the natural history and ethology of dogs and cats that are relevant to what and how we feed them. Dogs are scavengers by nature, as well as hunters, being more omnivorous than cats who have a lower tolerance and natural aversion for spoiled meat and other foods. After an estimated 100,000 years and more of being domesticated and living with humans, dogs adapted to a diet of leftovers from the human table, most of the protein (meat) being consumed by humans. As free-roaming animals in the community, dogs survived and adapted as omnivorous scavengers. This does not mean that modern dogs should be given poor quality food. But they may not tolerate a high protein diet, and as scavengers may do better being given 3-4 small meals a day instead of one large meal. Feeding a dog only one large meal daily may increase the chances of bloat and other less serious digestive problems. A very high protein diet may contribute to kidney disease, dysplasia and other health problems in certain individuals and breeds.

Cats have been domesticated for a much shorter time, and during that time they were still primarily kept to control rodents around the farm or homestead, and thus stayed close to their natural, carnivorous diet.

The transition from eating wild caught game/prey and later, the human left-overs from free-range farmed animals, and then more recently, conventionally raised 'factory' farmed animal parts and remains, has been nutritionally challenging for dogs and cats in the developed world. Of particular concern are high levels of saturated fats increasingly contaminated with dioxins and PCBs; omega 3 polyunsaturated fatty acid deficiencies and pro-inflammatory omega 6 excesses. Heavy metal contaminants like lead, copper, cadmium and arsenic in ground bone and organ parts, antibiotic, anabolic steroid and other veterinary and production drug residues, lipophilic pesticide contaminants in fatty tissues, along with mercury contamination in sea foods, pose additional health risks.

Domestic animals do adapt to diets that are sub-optimal, through natural selection, those who are free-ranging being sometimes able to compensate for nutritional deficiencies in what food is given to them, by hunting and scavenging.

The health consequences of under-nutrition and nutrient deficiencies have been fairly well documented over the years, while over-nutrition and its harmful consequences are more recent problems. Examples include too much protein in older animals, too many calories for sedentary pets, too many carbohydrates for cats and dogs, and too much protein in puppy hood for certain breeds like Labradors. Pups and adult dogs who are biologically adapted as scavenging aboriginal or 'pariah' dogs may be especially prone to the harmful consequences of over-nutrition when given the kinds of food that provide optimal nutrition for most dogs in Western society.

Feeding dogs and cats highly processed and variously denatured human food and beverage-industry byproducts, artificial additives, preservatives, and chemical supplements, is another biological challenge, and is not consistent with their dietary natural history. Also cats are not adapted, in terms of their thirst mechanism, to thrive on dry foods.

Dogs and cats are not always immediately adapted physiologically to a diet that consists entirely of raw whole foods. Transitioning to such a diet should always be gradual. The Precautionary Principle should also be exercised when introducing an animal to a complete or partial raw food diet. Raw beef and poultry products need to be handled with care, since modern intensive livestock production and centralized processing are responsible for frequent outbreaks of E. coli, Lysteria, Salmonella, and other forms of bacterial food poisoning in humans, and companion animals may also be affected. Thoroughly cooking ground meats before feeding is advisable. Solid chunks of meat should be scalded, or rinsed in cold running water before serving raw to dogs and cats. Raw pork should not be given because of the risk of Trichinosis, a parasitic disease, and other raw animal remains such as fish may also harbor transmissible parasitic and pathogenic organisms.

There is evidence that dogs and cats seek out their own natural dietary supplements as needed. They eat various grasses and certain herbs, and dogs especially enjoy deer and horse feces and sometimes eat soil with high mineral content, especially when anemic. Both dogs and cats will eat the entire carcass of small prey, which includes partially digested plant foods and bacteria (probiotics?) in the prey's digestive systems.

Dogs and cats kept confined indoors may be deprived of such natural dietary supplements and cannot exercise their "nutritional wisdom." Some consideration should therefore be given to this other aspect of dietary natural history, as by putting chopped barley or alfalfa sprouts in the animals' food, and by providing probiotics and digestive enzymes. More research is also called for in this area of natural organic supplements.

CHAPTER 13
Why Most Manufactured Pet Foods
Should Not be Fed to Dogs & Cats

Regardless of the largest ever pet food recall, in spring of 2007, that resulted in the poisoning and deaths of thousands of dogs and cats across North America, my answer to this question, unlike many of my veterinary colleagues, is that I have come to believe that dogs and cats should not be fed most manufactured pet foods as their main or only source of nutritional sustenance.

I have come to this conclusion because of the dramatic clinical improvement in dogs and cats suffering from a number of chronic, debilitating, and costly health problems once they have been taken off highly processed commercial pet foods and are given naturally formulated, organic whole food diets appropriate for their species, age, physical condition, and activity level.

Scientifically formulated, manufactured pet foods are packed with chemical supplements used to 'fortify', i.e. make up for deficiencies in the basic ingredients that are slaughter house and food and beverage industry waste byproducts, and other chemical additives to flavor/taste-enhance, stabilize, preserve, color and 'texturize' (appear like meat and gravy rather than a grey mush). According to a CNN News report on July 20, 2007, such supplements that are put into processed foods for human consumption as well as in to pet foods are not subject to any FDA inspection or oversight, and the government has no records as to country of origin of these additives/supplements.

Many micronutrients are destroyed by processing, excessive exposure to heat and/or water denatures proteins, destroying essential amino acids, vitamins C, thiamine, niacin, riboflavin, and some of the essential fatty acids. Acidification of the diet can destroy acid-sensitive micronutrients like vitamin K, biotin and B-12.

Acidification has been done for several years by pet food manufacturers to help control struvite crystal formation in the urine that becomes too alkaline when dogs and cats are fed high cereal diets. This can lead to the development of calculi/stones in the urinary tract that cause painful and even fatal urinary blockage. Such artificial alteration of the acidity/alkalinity of the animals' food can cause metabolic acidosis and kidney failure. These are common emergencies, along with urinary retention, in veterinary practice. Acidification of pet foods also resulted in an increased incidence of calcium oxalate uroliths/stones.

Oxidation/rancidification of pet foods and their ingredients during storage and transport is another problem. Most pet food manufacturers have recently phased out using BHA and BHT that were used for many years as preservatives in both human and pet foods. Animal tests have linked BHA to stomach and bladder cancer, and BHT to thyroid and bladder cancer. Pet food manufacturers now use 'mixed tocopherols' (a claimed source or form of vitamin E), citric acid, beta-carotene and Rosemary extract as preservatives. High levels of vitamin E, the most widely used antioxidant in pet foods today, can disrupt the activity of the other fat soluble vitamins, namely vitamins A, D and K, so these are often added as supplements to the formula, which is not without risk since vitamins A and D can be toxic at biologically excessive levels in the food.

There are additional chemical contaminants not listed on the pet food label that were associated with the production, processing, and preserving of the original sources of the primary ingredients like animal fat, chicken meal and corn meal, including pesticide residues, animal drugs, ethoxyquin (a known carcinogen) to prevent tallow from becoming rancid, and polyacrylamide used to coagulate slaughter house waste. Mercury compounds in fish products, and dioxins and PCBs in most animal byproducts are additional concerns, as is the lower nutritional value of conventionally grown crops compared to organically grown.

To claim that manufactured pet foods are scientifically formulated and are therefore safe and provide complete nutrition for growth and health maintenance is as incorrect as contending that genetically engineered crops and foods are 'substantially equivalent' to conventional crops and foods and are therefore as safe and as nutritious. The former claims have proven, year after year, to be patently false and misleading, as exemplified by the many animals becoming ill because of deficiencies in taurine and essential fatty acids, and from imbalances in calcium and phosphorus and essential trace minerals.

Pet food container labels include such statements as 'Animal feeding tests substantiate that this product provides complete and balanced nutrition for all life stages,' or 'for growth and maintenance.' The science supporting the pet food industry was based until recently not on veterinary nutritional science, but on the animal production science of livestock feed formulation that relies on simplistic ingredient analysis and formulation as per the 'Guaranteed Analysis' on pet food labels that shows the percentage of crude protein, fat, carbohydrate, fiber and ash. The list of supplements/additives is always longer than the list of the basic ingredients such as chicken meal, meat byproduct and corn meal.

Veterinary clinical nutrition is essentially applied after the fact, once feeding trials are conducted on basic low-cost ingredient formulations and then potential and reported health problems are corrected by the inclusion of various additives/supplements. Feeding trials to determine safety and nutritional values are not cost-effective and so are not done on a regular basis but should be with every new formulation and when ingredients from different sources are used.

In actuality, standardization in terms of quality can be better established for synthetic, manufactured chemical additives/supplements than for the basic food ingredients. Yet this is not without risk considering the recent recall of pet food containing toxic levels of Vitamin D that caused systemic calcinosis in cats. Standardization of supplement/additive amounts, in terms of the quantity added to each batch of manufactured pet food cannot be established without knowing what is in the basic food ingredients, and that can vary widely according to supplier, time in storage, degree of prior processing etc. Plant ingredients, often contaminated with aflatoxin and other toxic molds, can be deficient in iron, zinc, selenium, magnesium, vitamin A and C, and lysine, among other essential nutrients and high in phytoestrogens, endocrine disrupting agrichemicals, dioxins, and PCBs, the latter being a serious problem because of bioaccumulation in animal-derived food ingredients.

Aside from bacterial contamination, notably with Salmonella and E. coli, animal derived ingredients can throw off supplement calculations when high in calcium, a common result of de-boning; high in contaminants like mercury, lead, cadmium, and arsenic; deficient in essential fatty acids like omega 3, but high in omega 6; and deficient in zinc, selenium and magnesium. Fewer tests of primary ingredients would be needed for known-source and inspected, humane and organically certified producers and marketers of agricultural commodities for human and animal consumption. Tests on organic produce, both vegetable and animal-derived, have shown consistently higher levels of vitamins, trace minerals and other essential nutrients compared to conventionally grown crops.

The difference between naturally constituted whole foods and scientifically concocted manufactured pet foods can be seen on the pet food labels with a plethora of synthetic vitamins, amino acids and trace minerals of dubious nutritive value and origin (as from China) deemed essential because of the poor quality of lowest-cost basic ingredients, and because of the destruction/denaturing of essential nutrients due to processing, storage and cooking. Aside from the fact that major pet food companies are still selling predominantly cereal-based cat foods (e.g. combinations of corn meal, corn gluten meal, brewers rice, wheat, and soy flour), as 'complete and balanced nutrition for all life stages according to AAFCO animal feeding tests' which, for documented health reasons, is unethical, dog and cat foods can include the following non-nutritive additives:

Manufactured pet foods can contain humectants like sugar/ sucrose, corn syrup, sorbitol and molasses; antimicrobial preservatives like propionic, sorbic and phosphoric acids, sodium nitrite, sodium and calcium propionate and potassium sorbate; natural coloring agents like iron oxide and caramel, and synthetic coloring agents like coal-tar derived azo-dyes such as Yellow 5, Red 40, Yellow 6, and Blue 2; emulsifying agents used as stabilizers and thickeners, such as seaweed, seed, and microbial gums, gums from trees, and chemically modified plant cellulose like citrus pectin, xanthan and guar gum, and carrageenan; flavor and palatability enhances include 'natural' flavors, 'animal digest', and even MSG (monosodium glutamate); natural fiber like beet pulp, and miscellaneous additives like polyphosphates that help retain natural moisture, condition and texture of manufactured pet foods.

Red 2G food coloring has been identified by the European Food Standards Authority as a carcinogen, and other coal-tar and petrochemical-derived Azo dyes used as food (and beverage) coloring agents are now being re-evaluated.

Gimmicky additions to pet foods include marigold and chicory extract, and touting chicken byproduct meal as a 'source of chondriotin and glucosamine' in reality means that much of this ingredient is probably of low protein value because it contains a lot of cartilage and bone from the remains of ground up chicken parts not considered fit for human consumption.

It would be prudent for all pet food manufacturers, especially after the massive pet food recall in the U.S. in the spring of 2007 that resulted in the suffering of uncounted numbers of dogs and cats, to clearly indicate on the pet food container labels how they can be reached by pet owners and veterinarians with product related questions and concerns. Every new batch of untested pet foods containing either new ingredients or the same ingredients but from new sources should be appropriately numbered, and annual reports of any adverse food reactions should be available to veterinarians upon request, and filed with the appropriate governmental regulatory authority. All labels should also indicate the form of nutrient supplements, organic chelated minerals, for example, being better assimilated than inorganic minerals.

Cats are notorious for becoming addicted to dry foods, and such foods, generally condoned by veterinarians because they believe the manufacturers' claim that the food is scientifically formulated and balanced for health and maintenance, and helps keep cats' teeth clean, can result in several serious diseases, from obesity and skin problems to diabetes and urinary tract problems. (See Elizabeth Hodgkins, DVM, Esq, *Your Cat*, published by St Martin's Press, NY 2007 for further documentation).

Both dry and canned dog and cat foods contain ingredients that can cause food-allergy or hypersensitivity, and may also lack essential nutrients that lead to various skin and other health problems. But because most veterinarians believe in what the pet food manufacturers claim, (and recent graduates are no exception when one looks at the funds provided to State and private veterinary colleges by the pet food industry), they rarely suggest changing their sick animals' diet. Instead they practice iatrogenic medicine, first by endorsing the continued feeding of potentially harmful diets, then by prescribing potentially harmful drugs and costly special prescription diets that are all too often useless and highly unpalatable.

Following the initiative of drug companies, major pet food companies now also endow Chairs and fund departments, lectureships and student fellowships and prizes at every veterinary college in the US, and around the world in countries where profits are to be made.

It is no coincidence that one of the biggest American pet food manufacturers in the U.S. is now selling Pet Health Insurance policies.

As a more informed consumer populace says 'no' to junk/fast/convenience foods, so the days are numbered for the other agribusiness food and beverage industry subsidiary, namely the main-stream commercial pet food manufacturer, unless it chooses to meet the rising public demand for safe and nutritious food for all. And that, surely, would be an ethically enlightened business decision, since continued resistance to change, denial, lack of accountability, and defense of the status quo are ultimately counterproductive and self-defeating regardless of the $15 billion annual income enjoyed by U.S. pet food manufacturers. But public trust will be hard to regain after the debacle of the largest pet food recall ever in the U.S. in the Spring of 2007 of some 60 million containers bearing scores of different manufacturer and supplier labels, including all the big brand names, that left an estimated 8,500 dogs and cats dead, and harmed hundreds of thousands of others.

There is a new generation of commercial cat and dog foods, from raw to freeze-dried, canned to dry, that contain organically certified, whole food ingredients, properly formulated and balanced, (i.e., not loaded with cereal and meat industry byproducts), that are now appearing on grocery shelves, and being marketed by local and national supply networks. Also several good books are available for preparing home-made cat and dog food. This trend goes hand in hand with increasing consumer demand for organically produced, minimally processed foods as more health and environmentally conscious shoppers vote with their dollars and sense: And with veterinarians recognizing and the harmful consequences of most manufactured pet foods, and treating their animal patients accordingly.

The words of health and fitness guru ninety-six old Jack LaLanne are as relevant to what we eat ourselves as to what people feed to their cats and dogs. He asserts, quite simply, "If man makes it, don't eat it."

Pet Health & What We Eat & Feed Them

Let your food be your medicine and your medicine be your food—
    Hippocrates 460-377 BC
(An earlier version of this section was published in the *Journal of the American Holistic Veterinary medical Association*, vol.27, p 20-27, 2008)

The following review examines the thesis that many of the serious, chronic, and costly health problems seen today in companion animals that mimic diet-related medical conditions in the consumer populace are due primarily to high-calorie food commodities (corn, soy, wheat and rice), and livestock raised on these commodities becoming the basis of the US diet, displacing a wide range of health-supporting whole foods, (Ludwig and Pollack, 2009). This government-subsidized human, livestock, and pet food oligopoly is extremely pathogenic to the end-consumer, poisoning the environment and undermining all attempts to improve public health and an affordable and effective health care system.

Until relatively recent times, the role of diet and nutrition in preventing a host of diseases has been more a common sense given than a subject of scientific study. More and more health problems in humans and animals alike are being dramatically reversed or prevented by dietary changes. Over the past decade there has been a surge of research into the health benefits of certain nutrients, probiotics, prebiotics, and herbal and nutraceutical supplements. The vital importance of maintaining a healthy intestinal flora has been underscored time and again. Ironically, many of the health problems that afflict people and their pets have a common root-connection with highly processed convenience foods and so called fast foods and junk foods.

Many people are surprised when their cats turn out to be allergic to fish, but this should be no surprise because house cats were a desert dwelling species originally, and fish was obviously never part of their natural diet. This is the first clue to the potential hazards of 'foreign' or novel proteins in biologically inappropriate foods. We might also speak of culturally and racially inappropriate foods in the same breath, allergies in Caucasians not adapted to the Mesoamerican foods like peanuts or groundnuts; and cats and dogs allergic to corn, another Mesoamerican crop now playing a central role in the Western diet.

It is ironic that Wheaten terriers are severely allergic to wheat, 'the staff of life,' but like other terriers from England, oats, rye, barley, groats, potatoes, offal and rats were their staple foods for generations. Wheat is a relatively recent inclusion into the Western European diet. Dogs from the Middle-east may be better adapted to wheat, chick peas, goat and lamb in their diets, just as those from the Orient are better adapted to rice and soy products in their diets, as well as some fish and poultry and pork offal. Cats and dogs may or may not be 'adapting' respectively to corn, soy, and other pet food ingredients. 'Natural selection' cannot operate to eliminate those animals who, because of their genotypes, develop overt health problems later in life when fed biologically inappropriate commercial diets, because the breeding stock are bred when young and before such maladies are likely to develop. So generations after generation of animals are going to suffer, while those dogs and cats with different genotypes will fare much better.

These sweeping generalizations aside, the hazards of genetically inappropriate foods are now a major focus of pet food research and human medicine alike, but there will be little progress so long as genetically engineered crop varieties proliferate, and the agricultural food commodity industry continues to fail to control another group of toxins in grains and corn from entering the food chain, namely those of various molds. Aflatoxin in pet foods, especially dry foods, may be a cause of 'sub-clinical' or pre-disease conditions especially of the liver at low levels, and at higher levels result in all too frequent recalls when cats, dogs and other pets sicken and die.

What crops are grown, and how, and what farmed animals,

including farmed fish are fed, have a direct bearing on pubic health and the health of cats and dogs fed the byproducts of the Western diet. This will be examined more thoroughly below. But at this time of writing it is to be noted that the main-stream medical profession is beginning to acknowledge at last the enormous health costs and consequences, not only of essential mineral and vitamin deficient foods and hazardous supplements and additives like the neurotoxic Aspartame, and dog-killing artificial sweetener Xylitol, but of the Western diet itself. For instance, there is growing recognition of the essential fatty acid crisis, where our foods are too high in pro-inflammatory Omega 6 fatty acids, and deficient in Omega 3s.

Many informed nutritionists promote Omega 3s-rich organic butter, also high in conjugated linoleic acid and antioxidants, as is beef tallow/lard if from a grass-based rather than corn and soy based diet; also organic coconut oil (high in lauric acid) and other nut oils as healthier alternatives, including seed oils like grape and sesame in moderation because of lectin content. Organic butter and wild fish oils are best for cats, and for dogs and cats with kidney disease.

The recycling of much used multi-chain restaurant and food manufacturer cooking oil, high in Omega 6 essential fatty acids and deficient in Omega 3 essential fatty acids and linoleic acid — especially soy, palm, cotton seed, peanut, sunflower, safflower corn and canola — back into livestock feed and pet foods is a case in point. It has helped bring on this fatty acid crisis, as pets and people get fatter and sicker in many ways! America's industrial agri-science response of creating genetically engineered pigs with a higher than normal content of desirable fatty acids for the human food chain, has been patented — and is a patently absurd waste of public funds!

Most Common Health Problems

Veterinary Pet Insurance (VPI) has released its list of the top 10 medical conditions for which claims were submitted last year for dogs and cats. VPI received more than a million claims in 2009. The most common ailment in dogs? Ear infection, coming in at nearly 68,000 claims and an average cost of $100 per visit. And in cats? Lower urinary tract disease, with a total of 3,700 claims at an average cost of $260 per visit. Here's the complete list (Table 13-1):

Table 13-1. Common Health Problems in Dogs & Cats

Top conditions in dogs	Top Conditions in Cats
1. Ear infection	1. Lower Urinary Tract Disease
2. Skin allergy	2. Gastritis, or vomiting
3. Skin infection, or hot spots	3. Chronic renal failure
4. Gastritis, or vomiting	4. Hyperthyroidism
5. Enteritis, or diarrhea	5. Diabetes
6. Bladder infection	6. Enteritis, or diarrhea
7. Arthritis	7. Skin allergy
8. Soft tissue trauma	8. Periodontitis, or dental disease
9. Noncancerous tumor	9. Ear infection
10. Eye infection	10. Eye infection

In the above synopsis of the most common health problems posted by VPI, the conditions requiring veterinary attention, with few if any exceptions, could have been prevented and effectively treated, by diet alone, in my professional opinion, and in the opinion of other holistic veterinarians who practice integrative medicine.

Significantly, Dr. Cori Gross, a field veterinarian for VPI (cited on www. VPIpetinsurance.com), advocates feeding cats canned food to prevent lower urinary tract diseases. She expected to see arthritis, at # 8 for dogs, in the top 10 list for cats, since it is also common in cats. It is observed that owners are less likely to notice.

It may seem curious that obesity did not get onto the top 10 lists for dog and cat health problems, since this is an increasing concern for both species. The reason obesity is not included in the VPI list of illnesses is that they do not include it in the things they reimburse for. In addition, most veterinarians don't have an obesity program. VPI covers all the conditions that RESULT from obesity (diabetes, arthritis, etc.), but, like all the major human and pet insurance companies, does not cover preventive medicine (unless you want to call vaccination and flea prevention preventive care—and they are only included on their premium policies).

Dr. Gross is also quoted on the VPI website report as being surprised that there were not more dental claims for dogs. Dental problems, closely related to diet, are very common in dogs and cats and are often left untreated for too long, causing much suffering and long crippling, even fatal illness. These include kidney, liver and heart disease secondary to periodontal disease that afflicts, to varying degrees of severity, an estimated seventy five percent of the US dog population. This is the oral equivalent of AIDS that goes from halitosis to toxicosis, and can lead to similar symptoms of immune system impairment associated with chronic oral disease/dysbiosis.

In a subsequent phone conversation with Dr. Gross, she concurred with my observations, stating that "Many of these conditions could be prevented or minimized by a change in diet." The early onset in life of these health problems in both the human and companion animal populations raises the possibility of epigenetic maternal nutrition-triggered influences during pregnancy.

The high incidence of urinary calculi in dogs and cats and in children as young as four or five, the Type 2 diabetes epidemic in children and pets, and the epidemic of overweight and obese pets and similar metabolic-obesity syndrome in people, all point to poor dietary factors, especially highly processed, prepared 'convenience,' and fast foods as the primary cause.

In their 2008 pet health insurance disease incidence report, the VPI include the following list of the most common afflictions that affect both people and pets (in descending order of incidence): allergies; bladder infection; arthritis; diabetes; skin cancer; gum disease; acne; stomach ulcers; cataracts; laryngitis. Note; allergies were one of the top pet health insurance claims in 2008.

Behavioral Problems

Another possible diet-related health issue in children and companion animals entailing behavioral, affective, and cognitive impairment, often coupled with neuroendocrine disturbances and food allergies, has resulted in the use of more and more psychotropic drugs in pets and first graders. How else to deal with obsessively compulsive, aggressively impulsive, attention-impaired companion animals and school children, if no thought is given to what they are consuming, and may be consuming them? Excess quantities of Omega 6 fatty acids and Omega 3 fatty acids deficiency can play a major role in such afflictions. The high levels of glutamine, alanine, and taurine in the urine of aggressive dogs reported by veterinarian Dr. Karen Overall may be associated with high glutamate content in manufactured pet foods. (See below for further discussion).

Obesity and the Metabolic Syndrome

The main-stream pet food industry is as much to blame for this obesity epidemic as are those veterinarians who continue to see no connection between diet and the carnivore metabolic syndrome (CMS), as I prefer to call this condition. Highly processed cereal carbohydrates in the food cause an almost immediate 'sugar rush' every time the cat or dog eats.

High fructose corn syrup is used as a flavoring in some dog and cat food, and along with other sugars, as a browning and caramelizing agent, and especially in semi-moist package foods and treats (still laced with propylene glycol and azo-dyes), as a preservative. This sugar reaction damages the liver and the pancreas, resulting in the conversion of sugar into body fat in many animals, with or without diabetes and fatty liver disease. The 'sugar rush' and insulin surge (until the pancreas becomes exhausted) make many cats and dogs constantly hungry, so they quickly become obese. Owners think their animal companions love the dry food because they always want to eat it.

CMS entails much more systemic damage than simply storing fat. Animals who become overweight or obese primarily as a result of the kinds of manufactured foods they are fed, rather than simply being over-fed and under-exercised, are likely to develop a host of health problems. These include diabetes, arthritis, skin disease, pododermatitis (canine interdigital cysts), chronic inflammations and infections like cystitis, gingivitis, and otitis, heart and liver disease, hepatic lipidosis (also a recognized problem in obese children), lipomas and cancer. Poor nutrition can also lead to immune system impairment and increased susceptibility to infectious organisms and chemical allergens in the environment.

The Gluten Issue
Cereals contain natural opiates that could lead to addiction, but the high gluten content of cereals such as wheat, barley, oats and rye (with the exception of millet, buckwheat, brown rice and quinoa) can be problematic for both humans and their pets. Corn gluten meal, a protein derivative byproduct of processing, is in most pet foods. It is the biggest source of gluten for dogs and cats.

Gluten is used as a cheap protein ingredient in pet foods, and is especially unsuitable for obligate carnivores like cats. Gluten-sensitivity is associated with a host of illnesses arising, in part from the 'leaky gut' syndrome and intestinal dysbiosis (bacterial imbalance). These illnesses include allergies, chronic skin and digestive problems, malabsorption and nutrient deficiencies, Addison's disease, and epilepsy. Gluten-sensitive enteropathy is a recognized condition in some dog breeds such as Wheaten terriers and Irish setters.

High glutamate levels evident in many manufactured pet foods, along with monosodium glutamate that comes primarily from human food and beverage industry byproducts include soy protein, wheat gluten, whey protein, barley malt, natural beef flavoring, natural chicken flavoring, carrageenan, calcium caseinate, gelatin, textured and hydrolyzed protein (usually soy), yeast extract, pectin, 'seasonings' and 'natural' flavors. The fermented offal called 'meat digest' that is sprayed on dry pet foods to enhance palatability/addiction is likely to contain high levels of glutamate. (Note: monosodium glutamate is the anionic form of glutamic acid. Glutamine differs from glutamate in that it is formed from glutamate and ammonia by the enzyme catalyst glutamine synthetase.)

High glutamate levels from the cheap proteins put into pet foods and human junk food may play a significant role in a host of common diseases such as taurine deficiency disease, which caused an epidemic of blindness, heart disease and brain damage in cats until partially rectified. Differential uptake of taurine by gut bacteria, leaving less for the cat to absorb, may be part of the dysbiosis created by high cereal-content diets. More taurine is now put into manufactured pet foods because high glutamate levels block the uptake of the essential amino acid taurine. The spiking with taurine does nothing to stop the other harms of glutamate poisoning.

The 'Chinese Restaurant' syndrome is not just an acute MSG-induced headache, often with flushing, blood pressure elevation, sweating, tinnitus, and feeling full; there is also the after-shock of an increased and unexpected hunger that comes on soon after what was felt, initially, to be a long-satisfying meal. This reaction is often compounded by the high sugar and simple carbohydrate/starch content in Chinese entrées and in many snack and convenience foods that form the basis of the Western diet. The inclusion of sugars and starches in manufactured pet foods, like molasses, corn starch, and rice flour, needs to end.

Cats and dogs on many manufactured pet foods suffer the equivalent of the Chinese restaurant syndrome every day. They are always hungry, demanding food, and soon become, like junk-food addicted people, obese, diabetic, and more prone to allergies, thyroid disease, depression, irritability/aggression, seizures, Alzheimer's disease, hypertension, and a host of other disorders of body and mind. Excess glutamate in manufactured foods is a serious problem for all. So a complete or partial raw food diet would be preferable for dogs, cats and their owners too!

Humans and Pets Harmed by Lectins
Allergenic and hypersensitive reactions to various pet food ingredients are triggered especially by cereal grain gluten (wheat, barley and rye), more specifically by carbohydrate binding proteins called lectins, of which gliadin in gluten is one. Malnutrition and nutritional deficiency diseases

like anemia and osteoporosis—that the cocktail of synthetic vitamins, minerals, etc. in manufactured pet foods does not prevent—result after the intestinal wall is damaged by these glue-like lectins. Cow milk casein (the bovine equivalent of gluten, also used to make glue), and soy and corn gluten can be problematic for some animals and people too.

Damage to the digestive tract can also lead to dysbiosis—the overgrowth of potentially harmful bacteria and yeasts—, and to the so called 'leaky gut' syndrome. This occurs when the damaged intestinal wall allows the body to absorb much larger protein molecules than normal. Some of these, like the lectins in grains and beans like soy, could cause cell damage and set of a cascade of health problems in various organ systems, or trigger allergic reactions to these foreign proteins that in turn could lead to neuroendocrine and autoimmune diseases. Lectins have been linked in humans to infantile diabetes (especially from dairy products); to celiac disease, rheumatoid arthritis, and diseases of the kidneys, pancreas, adrenals (e.g. adrenal insufficiency), thyroid, and heart, and also may play a role in cancer, possibly by activating dormant viruses in the DNA of cells.

Many so called 'idiopathic' diseases in humans and their pets, from epilepsy to psoriasis, and arthritis to gingivitis, have been cured simply by dietary changes and supplements. Those treated conventionally with no changes in diet bear the harmful consequences of widely prescribed drugs such as prednisone, the NSAIDs, antibiotics, costly immuno-enhancers and suppressors, even psychotropic drugs for neurological and behavioral/ emotional problems such as depression, hyperactivity, and obsessive compulsive disorder.

Some breeds, races, and individuals are more susceptible than others to these nutrition- and diet-related health problems associated in particular with lectins, some of which can be neutralized by nutraceuticals such as glucosamine and oligosaccharides (like inulin and aloe vera liquid). Many with genetically-based intolerance may develop degrees of tolerance, but we do not know how many dogs and cats, as well as their owners, slip under the radar, at least for a few years, before sub-clinical malaise becomes evident dis-ease. Under holistic medical care, many afflicted people benefit from the so-called 'Paleolithic diet' that excludes high-lectin containing foods. The evident trend of many small pet food manufacturers to market grain, corn and soy-free cat and dog foods is a logical step and may do much to help eliminate many so called 'iatrogenic', diseases and autoimmune and chronic degenerative diseases in companion animals that have a species- or breed-specific, genetically based intolerance.

There is also the factor of soy bean ingredients used as a cheap source of protein being rich in phytoestrogens. These could contribute to endocrine disruption and play a role in obesity. Soy may be one of several significant factors in the current epidemic of hypothyroidism in dogs fed conventional pet foods. Before the advent of such foods, this condition was uncommon in most breeds.

Of course there are other factors to consider in the complex disease syndromes that we face today. These include a host of chemical contaminants especially in food, water and home environments, many of which are endocrine disruptors, and adverse reactions to vaccinations, over-use of same, along with 'preventive' drugs against fleas, ticks, heartworm and other parasites.

The interaction between nutrition and vaccination efficacy should be *underscored*, poor nutrition being associated with poor antibody responses to vaccinations. Some veterinarians therefore advocate giving anti- oxidant supplements and probiotics to animals a few days before they are to be vaccinated.

Allergies, Food Hypersensitivity, & Immune System

The dramatic increase in food-related allergic diseases and digestive problems in children and pets over the last decade may be linked to more and more foreign proteins, especially spliced-in lectins from other plants, in their diets that come from genetically engineered crops. Novel proteins in GM (genetically modified or engineered) crops and foods can act as allergens, notably the Bt-toxin in corn, and have been shown to have negative effects on every body organ and system in test animals.

The high incidence of skin allergies, and other suspected allergies associated with digestive disorders and inflammatory bowel disease in dogs and cats may well be caused or aggravated by novel proteins and other chemical contaminants, particularly herbicide residues, in GM ingredients in manufactured pet foods. Animal lab tests confirm this risk. I have seen a dramatic increase in these problems over the past decade in the thousands of letters I receive from cat and dog owners who read my syndicated column.

It is surely no coincidence that in Oct. 2008, the US Centers for Disease Control and Prevention reported an 18% increase in allergies from 1997-2007 in children under the age of 18 years. Some 3 million children now suffer from food or digestive allergies, their symptoms including vomiting, skin rashes, and breathing problems. They take longer to outgrow milk and egg allergies, and show a doubling of adverse reactions to peanuts.

Some animals, just like some people, develop allergic reactions to now widely used artificial scents (in kitty litter, air 'fresheners', and other synthetic and treated materials brought into the home environment), the volatile organic compounds in these materials, as well as various phthalates, (also in many plastic food and liquid containers) being recognized as potentially damaging to the immune and neuroendocrine systems. The issue of chemical synergism, where chemicals in combination become more toxic, raises the specter of synergism between such environmental pollutants, adulterants and contaminants present in the food and water. (Fluoride in water is of particular concern since it is associated with thyroid disease, bone cancer and other health problems, while chlorination is a trade-off between possible bacterial contamination and potential endocrine disruption from chlorine compounds).

Herbicides & Digestive System Bacterial Health
It is not widely understood that the digestive tract is not simply an organ system designed for the assimilation of food. It is our primary organ of defense against potentially harmful food and water-born toxins, viruses, bacteria, and other potentially harmful organisms. Integral to this lymphatic-intestinal defense system is the population of intestinal 'flora'—bacteria and other microorganisms — that are symbiotic, having a symbiogenetic (mutually enhancing) relationship with the cells of the gut that recognize them immunologically as eubiotic enteric residents (i.e. helpful resident organisms). This is an adaptive response because these enteric bacteria act as a defense against invasive organisms, and provide the cells with various nutrients essential to the health and functional integrity of the rest of the body, much as the mycorrhyzas do around the roots of plants.

Agrichemicals, especially the herbicide residues in GM crops and their even more toxic breakdown products, when digested by humans and their pets, could cause a host of health problems if the normal gut flora is harmed. If this healthy, disease-preventing, nutrition-providing, and immune system-supporting population of symbiotic bacteria in the intestines is disrupted, nutritional deficiencies, overwhelming bacterial infection (Clostridia in dogs, for example), increased susceptibility to 'allergies', and other neuroendocrine and metabolic changes may ensue. These health problems have been linked in recent research to imbalances in the intestinal bacterial population where some species of bacteria come to dominate. This condition of dysbiosis is compounded by the over-prescribing by doctors of antibiotics and their wholesale use in livestock feed. Recent evidence that antibiotic residues in livestock manure can be absorbed by food crops raises another factor in the genesis of intestinal dysbiosis. What we are doing to our digestive system bacterial flora and to that of our companion animals mirrors what we have done to the beneficial microorganisms of the living soil that in turn affects the health and nutritive value of crops.

The most widely used herbicides sprayed on GM (genetically modified or engineered) herbicide-resistant cotton, corn, soybean and canola, such as Monsanto's Roundup (glyphosate) and Bayer's Ignite (glufosinate), can also have toxic effects on the body. Glyphosate may be an endocrine disruptor, and in test animals has caused elevation of some liver enzymes and calcium oxalate crystals to form in the urine, along with inflammatory changes in the kidneys and lower urinary tract.

As predicted over a decade ago, Monsanto's herbicide Roundup, (glyphosate) now used world-wide has resulted in the emergence of herbicide-resistant weeds, from Australia and Brazil to over 22 states in the US where Roundup-resistant crops of corn, soybeans and cotton are infested with invasive herbicide-resistant plants. Aside from concerns that farmers have applied more of this herbicide to attempt to control these invasive weeds, and the fact that GM crops sprayed with Roundup show defective uptake of essential nutrients such as magnesium and iron, Ag. Biotech companies are developing new GM crops with resistance to other herbicides, according to a report in *Acres U.S.A.* (July, 2010, p 8). Monsanto already has a patented GM corn resistant to glyphosate and glufosinate and is developing crops resistant to an older herbicide, dicamba; Bayer is selling corn and cotton resistant to glufosinate; Syngenta is developing soybeans tolerant of its Callisto herbicide, and Dow Chemical is developing corn and soybeans resistant to 2, 4-D, a component of the infamous Agent Orange used in the herbicidal warfare program in Vietnam.

Glufosinate can inhibit glutamine uptake. Deficiency of this amino acid is linked with bowel/digestive problems, impaired immune function, and possibly obesity due to increased appetite. It may be no coincidence that glutamine is widely prescribed for pets with 'leaky gut' syndrome and inflammatory bowel disease, and probiotics and prebiotics (like inulin and oligofructose) prescribed to help animals with allergies and other related health problems. Probiotics may also be of benefit in cases of pancreatitis, urinary tract infections, and oxalate uroliths.

Dysfunctional Agriculture, Hazardous Foods

We should not be surprised that there are so many nutrition-related health problems when we look at the soil that is used to produce food commodities that are not organically certified. As one California farmer told me some thirty years ago, 'Farmers today just use the soil to prop up their plants. Then they pour on the chemical fertilizers that they must, because they killed the soil with pesticides." Petrochemical-based agriculture has made our life-sustaining soil deficient in microorganisms that provide vital nutrients to the plants—and so our staple foods are also nutrient-deficient, especially in essential trace minerals and antioxidants like magnesium, zinc, and selenium.

Dead soil means no food without chemical fertilizers, herbicides, nematodicides, fungicides, insecticides, agricultural biotechnology's genetically engineered, cloned, and patented 'improved' varieties of crops and animals, with a frosting of USDA- & FDA-regulated food irradiation. While denying that Mad Cow Disease could be an endemic problem in US cattle, it is notable that the FDA prohibited the inclusion of brain and spinal chord in pet foods (the primary source of prions responsible for this neurological disease in cattle, pets and people), soon after the exposé of 'downer cow' cruelty at a California cattle handling and slaughter plant in early 2008.

Studies have shown that crops from organically certified producers, along with the meat and milk from farmed animals fed organic feed and allowed to graze on organically improved soils, contain far more essential nutrients than conventionally produced foods (refer to J. Cooper in Notes). And they suffer from far fewer viral and bacterial diseases which pose a serious public health concern today because of the intensive, concentrated animal production systems of the poultry, dairy and meat industry's 'factory farms.'

The billions of pounds of offal that is recycled into pet food and farm animal feed is the bedrock of the main stream pet food industry. But it is a hazardous waste. Bacterial contamination, as with Salmonella, can be so difficult to control that Mars Petcare decided to permanently close one of its pet food manufacturing facilities in Everson, Pa in 2008 because the entire plant could not be effectively sanitized. There had been repeated recalls of contaminated dry dog and cat food, associated with nearly 80 reported cases of human illness.

Offal includes condemned carcasses, inedible animal parts and trim that after processing are labeled meat meal, by-product meal and meat and bone meal "by-products." Being presumed heavily contaminated with harmful bacteria, offal is therefore subjected to high temperature and pressure sterilization and then slow cooking to evaporate off all moisture. The resultant solid is ground into a meal of essentially heat-denatured protein of little nutritive value. It loses more amino acids by evaporation, and others by cross-linkage into an indigestible product. Beef byproducts have less protein than chicken byproducts, and the actual digestible protein is significantly lower than the calculated 'protein' content of the manufactured dry dog and cat foods.

Time for Change

There is already a rush-to-market special and expensive, prescribed diets to help obese pets lose weight, along with an approved prescription-only diet pill for obese pets. Many veterinarians see this as a legitimate, profit-making business. There is a plethora of special prescription diets to help pets with a host of illnesses, such as allergies and digestive and urinary tract problems. But compared to simply transitioning cats and dogs onto a more biologically appropriate, whole-food diet with specific supplements and health restoring nutraceuticals as needed, these costly manufactured diets are of very limited value. Their scientific validity and medical efficacy are also questionable, especially the low-cal, high fiber weight loss formulations.

The veterinary profession is as yet behind, rather than leading, as it ought, the human medical profession, in addressing a host of health problems arising from manufactured pet foods, in part because of its ties to industry as an organized profession, colleges of which a richly endowed by the pet food industry: and in part because of indoctrination as students, that manufactured pet foods are scientifically formulated, animal tested, and provide complete and balanced nutrition for the health and maintenance of cats and dogs. There is much more to the basic ingredients and misleading terminology on the bag and can labels of these main-stream, main-street pet foods that the public trusts, no thanks to professional dog and cat performance events and other dog and cat shows, local, national, and international, that the pet food industry helps underwrite!

Commercial pet foods that people buy are a major factor in this obesity epidemic as well as a host of other health problems that are in part due to ignorance, overfeeding, and sheer convenience; and to the belief, shared, it would seem, by many veterinarians, that high cereal diets are not a significant contributing factor. Yet once informed, many pet owners will readily even cook home-prepared, wholesome, biologically appropriate meals for their animal companions, and attest to the almost immediate benefits observed in their animals' demeanor and vitality.

Fortunately, new approaches and solutions are on the horizon. This necessitates an understanding of how nutrients act and interact at the molecular level. Accordingly, nutrition research has shifted from epidemiology and physiology to molecular biology and genetics. Diets for animals should be designed and tailored to the genetic profile of individuals in order to optimize physiological homeostasis, disease prevention and treatment, and promote desired athletic, obedience or reproductive performances.

For example, a series of specialized semi-moist canned pet food formulas containing all human grade and organic food ingredients is now in clinical trials in Italy. These diets act as cleansing foods for the bowel and specific organs (e.g. liver and kidney) of pets with sub-acute and chronic illnesses. The specific needs of these animals are determined by applying the principle of nutrigenomics, where optimal nutrition can be designed based on an individual's unique genetic makeup or genotype. The resulting food formula is termed the "molecular dietary signature," and is formulated to restore the animal to health.

The Codes of Practice for the Welfare of Cats and of Dogs established by the UK Government's DEFRA (Department of Environment, Food and Rural Affairs) opens up pet owners to prosecution under the Animal Welfare Act (potentially facing up to 12 months in jail and a fine of up to 20,000 pounds sterling) if they allow their animals to become overweight/obese.

This may help veterinarians and pets' care-givers to work together to solve the problem of feline and canine obesity—DEFRA's Cat document clearly states cats are carnivores. This should mean that cereal-based cat foods will soon be off the shelves. So I would heartily endorse similar animal welfare legislation in the US and other countries that indirectly induces the public to be more responsible and support better farming methods and more nutritious prepared and convenience foods for their pets and for themselves.

It is time for a revolution in agriculture and consumer choices and habits. According to Business Week (August, 2008), two thirds of adult Americans are either overweight or obese, along with 23 million children.

This food health crisis cannot be denied any longer by those who claim to regulate agriculture, the food and beverage industries, and allow the mass poisoning of people and their pets with erroneously considered safe and nutritious basic ingredients, like corn, wheat, soy, dairy products and by-products. In these basic food commodities are metabolism and endocrine-disrupting ingredients, like corn fructose syrup, wheat and soy gluten, and certain cow milk immune-system disrupting glycoproteins. The public heavily subsidizes this agribusiness food industry with billions of dollars in government subsidies and price supports, indirectly underwriting its own demise—and nemesis.

Conclusions

The above documented concerns about manufactured pet foods are not meant to imply that all manufacturers do not care enough about dogs and cats to really become part of the solution. By 'solution', I mean becoming a creative participant in the food and agriculture revolution like those 'green' pet food companies and other pet product manufacturers and suppliers profiled by the author.

It is no coincidence that the Western diet, based on highly processed components of corn, soy, and cereal grains, and on the diary, meat and poultry products from animals fed these food commodities, should result in several recently identified, endemic health problems that are mirrored by cats and dogs fed the byproducts of this diet. The pork, poultry, egg, dairy, and beef industries, along with the prepared foods, beverage, and candy industries, use companion animals as highly profitable waste-recyclers. The irony is inescapable, considering the fact that these sectors of agriculture receive the greatest government support in subsidies and incentives, all at taxpayers' expense since these are public funds. But they are not being spent on the public good when we calculate the enormous health and environmental costs of the Western diet; and not to forget the horrendous existence of the animals down on the factory farm and feedlot.

Consumers and health-care providers alike are more widely realizing the connection between diet and the prevention and alleviation of a host of complex, so called degenerative, auto-immune, and idiopathic diseases that are in turn recognized as being brought on by other factors in addition to nutrition, or lack thereof. The so called pluri-causal, multifactor nature of such diseases makes it challenging to identify and control causal agents. But as evidence-based medicine affirms, often most effective treatment comes through attention to dietary factors.

With a burgeoning human population and growing social unrest with shortages of food, water, land and fuel, such a revolution—that includes the adoption of organic, low-input, sustainable farming methods and a reduction in meat production and consumption by many — is as vital to global food security as it is to national security and progress in public health.

The more that pet food companies obtain food ingredients from organic and alternative, sustainable sources rather than from conventional ones that rely on pesticides, cruel livestock and poultry confinement systems, and 'cheaper' imported crop and food-products and supplements, the more 'green' they become. It is enlightened self-interest for pet owners to support this food and agriculture revolution in their market choices for their pets and for themselves.

Postscript
Veterinarian-Formulated Recipes for Healthy and Sick Dogs and Cats
Balance IT® software and supplements, designed and supported by board certified veterinary nutritionists, help pet lovers and veterinarians acquire customized home-cooked diets that are complete and balanced. The Balance IT® Pet Lovers and Vet Express sites, found at www.balanceit.com, provide fast and easy tools for both healthy pets and pets with medical conditions. There are hundreds of different home-cooked diet formulations that can be individually calculated specifically for a pet's daily caloric needs. Recipes using both Balance IT® supplements and a combination of over-the-counter human supplements are available.

Tel:1-888-3Homemade (1-888-346-6362) (within the United States) Mailing address: Balance IT® Customer Support, DVM Consulting, Inc. 606 Peña Drive, Suite 700 Davis, CA 95618

Eat grain and suffer the consequences link: http://wideturn.com/ Holdingdirectory/CarbEating/fatthincarbs.htm

A few pages copied out of an 1891 encyclopedia (*The National Cyclopedia in 3 Volumes: A Dictionary of Useful and Practical Information For The Farm, Home And School*, by Hon. Jonathan Periam, Chicago, IL, R.S.Peale Co) illustrates how animals fed carbohydrates develop entirely different fat patterns and weaker bones than animals fed a more natural diet. This research done by W.A. Henry, Director of the Experiment Station, Wisconsin University, showed that pigs fed a high carbohydrate diet (corn—high in starch and low in protein) had:

1. Extensive development of fat, not only below the skin, but among the muscles
2. The muscles failed to develop to their normal size

3. Abnormally small amount of hair and thin skin
4. Spleen, liver and kidneys are abnormally small
5. Amount of blood in the body is greatly reduced
6. Strength of bones reduced by up to one half!

(The above list reads like a description of many dogs and cats we see today with their obesity, weak muscle tone, ruptured ligaments, orthopedic problems, and skin, hair, liver and kidney deficiencies.)

The author writes "... we may conclude that a system of feeding which robs the hog of half his blood and half the natural strength of his bones, and produces other violent changes, is a most unnatural one, and must, if persisted in, end in giving us a race of animals which will be unsatisfactory to all concerned. From the parents thus weakened, must come descendants that will fall easy victims to disease and disaster."

The author gratefully acknowledges the editorial work and content critique provided by cat-owner and rescuer Robin Scott, MD, and by veterinarians W. Jean Dodds, DVM, John B. Symes, DVM, and Nancy Scanlan, DVM, CVA, MSFP.

CHAPTER 14
Genetically Engineered & Modified Live Virus Vaccines: Public Health & Animal Welfare Concerns

By way of introduction to this critical review, I wish to make it clear at the onset that I am not opposed to the judicious use of vaccines. My approval is conditioned on the proviso that the deployed vaccines have high levels of proven safety and effectiveness for each species upon which they are used, and requires that they become part of an integrated, holistic health care and disease prevention program. When used as a sole therapy, vaccines do not constitute an effective preventive medicine regime. The myth of infectious and contagious diseases having a single cause—the infective organism—is at long last being abandoned as other co-factors are now being more widely recognized, extending the narrow view that developing a specific vaccine is all one requires to reduce the morbidity and mortality of a given disease.

As a veterinarian I am concerned about the consequences of the widespread dissemination of modified live virus (MLV) and genetically engineered (GE) virus strains through the mass vaccinations of humans, livestock and poultry, and in-house companion animals. Some GE vaccines have been widely used in several countries in bait to stop rabies in foxes, jackals, and other wild carnivores. These vaccines all contain live viruses, and supposedly weakened attenuated or inactivated strains recombined, like the pox virus which is used as an infective carrier, [or] spliced with an attenuated strand of rabies virus DNA. In a different context, this is akin to the Cauliflower mosaic virus that is used as a carrier of engineered genes in GE crops conferring herbicide tolerance and the manufacture of insecticidal proteins (Bt in corn). But there is one big difference. The aim of vaccination is to trigger an antibody immune response to the antigens in the vaccine. A poor response could lead to a case of the actual disease from the vaccine or vaccine failure, just as immunologic over-reaction (via aggressive anti-self antibody production) could mean death to the recipient.

In the US Government's Agriculture Fact Book 98, the Animal and Plant Health Inspection Service "regulates the licensing and production of genetically engineered vaccines and other veterinary biologics. These products range from diagnostic kits for feline leukemia virus to genetically engineered vaccines to prevent pseudorabies, a serious disease affecting swine. — Since the first vaccine was licensed in 1979, a total of 79 genetically engineered biologics have been licensed; all but 20 are still being produced. More than a half-century ago, there were perhaps a half a dozen animal vaccines and other biologics available to farmers. Now there are 2,379 active product licenses for these animal vaccines and other biologics and 110 licensed manufacturers." (1)

Hundreds of thousands of cats have been injected with a nonadjuvanted recombinant rabies vaccine spliced with the canary pox virus used as a 'vector.' According to Meeusen et al (2007), vectored vaccines are genetically modified organisms that have the genes responsible for encoding the desired antigens incorporated into the genetic code of a 'carrier' organism. The vector is noninfectious to the recipient and transmits the desired immunizing DNA/gene to a susceptible cell where the antigens are produced and presented to immune cells. The vector with the hybridized DNA is also called a chimera—having genes of two or more unrelated agents. The common vectors are capripox and canarypox viruses, adenoviruses and flaviviruses. These vaccines stimulate both antibody and cell-mediated antibody and, coincidentally, immunize with one dose. One concern is that repeated vaccinations may result in immunity to the vector virus eliminating its ability to infect/transmit the desired genes to the immune system. Currently, several vectored vaccines are used in companion animals.

Some genetically engineered viral vaccines consist of chimera viruses that combine aspects of two infective viral genomes. One example is the live Flavivirus chimera vaccine against West Nile virus (WNV) in horses (PreveNile), registered in the United States in 2006. The structural genes of the attenuated yellow fever YF-17D backbone virus have been replaced with structural genes of the related WNV. Chimera avian influenza virus vaccines have been produced on a backbone of an existing, attenuated Newcastle disease virus vaccine strain to protection against wild-type influenza virus as well as against Newcastle disease virus.

DNA vaccines are also being developed that consist of gene segments of infectious organisms. They are injected directly into cells for the production of the desired immunizing antigens. Intradermal injectors are used to deliver the DNA directly to the dendritic cells of the dermis. This system induces antibody and cell-mediated immunity with a single injection and provides prolonged immunity. A DNA vaccine is being tested for feline leukemia virus. A DNA vaccine licensed with the USDA has been developed to protect horses against viremia caused by WNV. This WNV infection, caused by a flavivirus belonging to the Japanese encephalitis virus complex, is enzootic in parts of Africa and Asia. It was first detected in 1999 in the US in an outbreak involving birds, horses, and humans in New York, subsequently spreading rapidly to many states.

I was particularly concerned by research being conducted at Philadelphia's Thomas Jefferson University Jefferson Vaccine Center under the direction of a Dr. Matthias J. Schnell who co-authored a scientific paper entitled "Rabies virus-based vectors expressing human immunodeficiency." The following is the Center's own synopsis of the research and development that is underway at that institution:

Research interests of the laboratory are the development of novel vaccines and viral pathogenesis.

Vaccines: Our laboratory develops Rhabdovirus-based [Rabies] vectors as vaccines against other infectious diseases. We are particularly interested in using molecular adjuvants and other molecules to enhance antigen-specific immunity and manipulate and retarget immune cells.

Using different molecular approaches, we perform detailed studies of highly attenuated RVs expressing HIV-1 or SIV genes and analyze their immunogenicity in mice. Our most promising HIV vaccine candidates are currently being analyzed in a monkey model for AIDS.

Other approaches include using genetically modified RV G proteins or RV capsids to carry antigens of other pathogens as vaccines against Anthrax and Botulism. We also seek to develop safer and more potent RV vaccines for wildlife and humans.

Pathogenesis: We are interested in understanding the interaction of rabies with the infected host at the molecular level. The molecular mechanism of rabies virus pathogenesis is not well understood, and our research analyzes the different functions of the rhabdoviral proteins (e.g. rabies virus) and their interactions with host proteins and the immune system.

Current projects are directed toward understanding:

• RV virus neurotropism and neuroinvasiveness: The transport of RV within neurons and the interaction of the RV phosphoprotein and glycoprotein with host proteins (receptors and transporter molecules)

• Immune responses of wild-type RV and RV-based vectors in the infected host (innate and adaptive)

GE virus developers Dongming Zhou, Ann Cun, Yan Li, and co-workers with Philadelphia's Wistar Institute, posted on line on June 22, 2006, (ARTICLE doi:10.1016/j.ymthe.2006.03.027) a report entitled "A Chimpanzee-Origin Adenovirus Vector Expressing the Rabies Virus

Glycoprotein as an Oral Vaccine against Inhalation Infection with Rabies Virus." Their summary reads as follows:

Rabies has the highest fatality rate of all human viral infections and the virus could potentially be disseminated through aerosols. Currently licensed vaccines to rabies virus are highly effective but it is unknown if they would provide reliable protection to rabies virus transmitted through inhalation, which allows rapid access to the central nervous system upon entering olfactory nerve endings. Here we describe preclinical data with a novel vaccine to rabies virus based on a recombinant replication-defective chimpanzee-origin adenovirus vector expressing the glycoprotein of the Evelyn Rokitniki Abelseth strain of rabies virus. This vaccine, termed AdC68rab.gp, induces sustained central and mucosal antibody responses to rabies virus after oral application and provides complete protection against rabies virus acquired through inhalation even if given at a moderate dose.

(These researchers used rodents, dogs, and primates in their research, and cultures of chicken fibroblasts).

This is a brief sample of the kind of vaccine research and development that is now going on world-wide. The use of recombinant replication-defective, vectored vaccines that express the proteins of rabies virus raises several issues, and comes close on the heels of using modified adenoviruses, herpesviruses and pox viruses as delivery systems for foreign antigens in livestock and poultry vaccines, and in bait to vaccinate and immuno-contracept wildlife (For details see OIE/world Organization fro Animal Health, Manual of Diagnostic tests and Vaccines for Terrestrial Mammals, 2008. www.oieint/eng/normes/mmanual/A_00099.htm).

In July 2009, the World health Organization reported several outbreaks in children of a mutated strain of poliomyelitis, identified as causing paralysis, originating from children who had been given the oral, modified live vaccine that they shed in their urine and feces, which forseeably infected unvaccinated children. Oral vaccination of red foxes against rabies in Ontario Canada, using a modified live virus vaccine in bait (often distributed from airplanes) has actually caused rabies in red foxes, raccoons, striped skinks and domestic animals (such as a bovine calf), according to Fehiner-Gardiner et al (2008).

Revisiting Vaccination Needs & Safety

The first vaccine was Edward Jenner's cow pox (vaccinia) that gave protection to a related human virus, small pox (variola) when injected into the skin. This practice of dispensing a mild infection in the form of a vaccine, to give protection against a more virulent, natural strain, is an ancient one. Masai and other African herders would make small incisions on healthy cattle's thighs and shoulders and then rub in a paste that included the secretions from sores of infected animals suffering from diseases like rinderpest, a virus closely related to measles and canine distemper viruses.

Jenner's discovery was a rare instance of cross-resistance, since subsequent vaccines did not have a less harmful related virus to use, but instead were usually composed of killed organisms of the same natural infective virus or bacterium to induce an immune response. A few safe and effective vaccines were developed to give protection from tetanus and diphtheria using the inactivated toxins from these bacteria.

More recently, weaker, so called attenuated, modified live virus (MLV) strains of the same species have been developed that ideally trigger specific antibodies and an immune system 'memory' to enable recipients to fight off infection. Immunocompromised individuals might get the disease from the actual MLV. In July 2006, Fort Dodge Animal Health recalled about 330,000 doses of a MLV rabies vaccine after a quality-assurance test indicated an issue with the duration of protection. The company confirmed one dog contracted rabies after receiving a dose from Serial 873113A of its Rabvac 3 TF vaccine. A statement from Fort Dodge added that the primary reason a vaccinated animal would contract the disease is because of a poor immune response. But, this does raise a red flag over the potential risks of widespread dissemination of modified live virus vaccines.

Until recently, most vaccines were given by injection, a route that was actually abnormal and possibly problematic, especially when adjuvants like mercury and aluminum were included in the antigen cocktail. Safer, more natural routes are via ingestion or inhalation, and are the focus of new vaccine research and development, especially for use in farmed animals in confined housing systems. But since natural infectious viruses tend to mutate, the strain used in the vaccine may not prove effective, or may give incomplete protection so that the recipient becomes a carrier or succumbs to the new infection.

Already we have seen MLV vaccines infect nontarget recipients, like nursing infants via the milk of recently vaccinated mothers. Some virologists believe that the feline distemper or panleukopenia virus mutated and crossed over from cats, or from some unidentified wild carnivore, to become canine parvovirus in dogs. There is now a strain of canine parvovirus (CPV) that can infect cats with a similar disease. Vaccines can be contaminated by other virus strains, abortions and deaths being reported in pregnant bitches receiving a commercial canine parvovirus vaccine inadvertently contaminated with blue tongue virus of sheep.

In-field Problems with Vaccines

The interactions between administering and receiving vaccinations and existing viral infections in animal populations can be complex and have harmful outcomes. Wildlife biologist Dr Roger Burrows (personal communication, May 13, 2009) writes that "Lions in Serengeti National Park (SNP), followed by those in the Masai Mara of Kenya, died like flies in 1994 from a new strain of canine distemper (CD). This followed a period 1992-94 when domestic dogs of agropastoralist/ farmers to the west, and Masai pastoralists dogs to the east of the SNP boundaries were being experimentally vaccinated against rabies during a vaccination trial." The same new strain of CD in the rabies vaccinated domestic dogs was subsequently found in the lions and was then found to have caused the death from CD of most of a captive colony of wild dogs (Lycaon pictus) in Mkomzai Game Reserve in Tanzania in 2000-2001—these wild dogs had been vaccinated against CD (using an inactivated strain developed for North Sea Seals!).

Following this, in 2007 the same new CD strain was for the first time identified in free living African wild dogs in Maasai areas to the east of SNP where mass vaccinations of local domestic dogs were being carried out against CD, CPV and rabies. The outbreak confirmed in one large wild dog pack was associated with high mortality of this highly endangered canid species.'

When local breeds of domestic dogs around Serengeti National Park (SNP) and the Masai Mara of Kenya were vaccinated against rabies and then soon after succumb to a virulent outbreak of CD it would seem to indicate that the rabies vaccinations caused some immunosuppression and thus increased susceptibility to CD. Attenuated vaccines should not be given to stressed and immunocompromised animals or humans.

Giving multivalent vaccines such as attenuated CD and CPV together could also be problematic, where one could make the other revert to a more virulent form due to the kind of reaction by the recipient to the other vaccine. Sensitization may occur following vaccination, and subsequent vaccinations could cause an acute inflammatory reaction, the so called cytokine storm, which could be fatal.

Vaccine Adjuvants

The inflammatory response to vaccinations, for which adjuvants have been blamed, is associated with the development of injection-site fibrosarcomas in cats and also dogs.

While there is a move toward developing adjuvant-free vaccines in order to minimize harmful side-effects (such as vaccine hypersensitivities, and mercury exacerbating preexisting autoimmune disease), adjuvants are still widely used. They are thought to enhance the immune response for small protein and glycoprotein antigens that elicit a weak immune response alone, by direct stimulation of the immune innate response (inducing local inflammatory reactions and stimulating the nonspecific proliferation of lymphocytes).

Aluminum salt and water/oil emulsions adjuvants are used in food animal vaccines, but can lead to granulomas developing at injection sites. Particulate or microsphere adjuvants are in limited veterinary usage in companion animal vaccines. They are made of biodegradable polymers that allow for a slow release of the antigen to the immune system.

Immunostimulatory complexes, (ISCOMS) are being developed and have been introduced into companion animal vaccines. They consist of a complex matrix of saponins, phospholipids and cholesterol incorporating the selected antigen. Their particulate structure enhances their interactions with antigen processing cells. ISCOMS tend to localize in lymph nodes draining the injection site prolonging the immune response, and can be administered at mucosal surfaces enhancing local antibody responses. Glycoside products, called Quill A from the Chilean soap bark tree, and saponins are used in some companion animal vaccines. Being quite toxic, these adjuvants require extensive purification to minimize toxicity. Squalene, a hydrocarbon triterpene, normally present in the human body as well as in shark liver and wheat germ, is used in conjunction with DL-a-tocopherol and polysorbate 80 as an adjuvant in flu and other vaccines (See Novartis MF59 and GlaxoSmithKline AS03 and AS 05). Injected squalene is suspected to cause a chronic inflammatory immune response in some individuals and may induce lupus antibodies and autoimmune arthritis.

The widely used vaccine preservative, Thimerosal, is a mercury-based compound that may damage DNA, neurons and T-cells.

Viruses Evolve & Mutate
Now that we have the new influenza viral strain, which on its evolutionary journey in pigs and poultry has killed wild birds, humans, dogs, and cats, we should honor the nature of viruses. And most importantly, we should not fight them with vaccine cocktails of antibodies with or without adjuvants, which can make recipients extremely ill, and even die. The latest influenza viral strain A/H1N1, isolated in human patients in the US, has a genetic sequencing indicating recombination of North American swine

influenza, human influenza, avian influenza, and Eurasian swine influenza virus.

The entire field of vaccinology and vaccine development, which appeals to and has attracted many brilliant scientists, is fraught by a reductionist paradigm that equates vaccinations with preventive medicine, rather than seeing it as a last resort at best, or a response in contexts where alternative methods of disease prevention and control have been tried and failed, e.g., sanitation).

The environmental and ecological consequences affecting interspecies balance, where modified live vaccines may be transferred horizontally as well as vertically and where one or more species and particular at-risk individuals, identified as those who are already immuno-compromised by stress, malnutrition, and infection, which may put other species and individuals at risk due to population disruptions, are not being considered in the decision to vaccinate. Or else the consequences of vaccination are simply dismissed. In many instances, mild viral infections are often best treated symptomatically and nutraceutical supplements given as preventatives, rather than run the risk of vaccinosis which could be for life and cause much suffering and expense.

The genetic—individual, familial, sub-species (or hybrid and selected breed or race) and species—represent important biotical variables in vaccine risks and benefits, and are now gaining some belated attention. But the epigenetic effects and transgenerational consequences of introducing live vaccines into human and animal (domestic and wild) populations have yet to be significantly addressed as representing potentially one of the greatest long-tem risks—far outweighing any benefits except to their manufacturers and dispensers.

Application of the precautionary principle is clearly called for, along with a vigorous bioethical evaluation, not simply to assess risks and benefits, and safety and effectiveness, but for real need and in-context determination, instituting the application, wherever appropriate, of alternative disease-prevention measures. These alternatives include improved housing and humane treatment of animals raised for food; better husbandry of free-range livestock and poultry to control diseases spread to wildlife (and vice-versa); not allowing pet cats and dogs to roam free, and community spay-neuter programs; improved shelter, nutrition, sanitation, clean water; and, socio-economic security incentives to facilitate the acceptance of family planning in many human communities around the world. In the developed world we should not be surprised when pig and poultry-specific viruses mutate under certain conditions, as in pig, poultry and rabbit factory farms, to become infectious to humans, cats, dogs and wildlife.

Vaccinoses Overlooked

Viruses are clearly an 'indicator' species reflecting their hosts' quality and kind of life. Repeated mass inoculations of people and their domestic animals can indirectly foster the selective evolution of other pathogens, or more virulent mutations, especially when the consequences of such 'public health' measures are not fully considered and addressed, such as within ever-increasing population numbers and concentrations/densities. This means no end to business for investors and vaccine and drug manufacturers.

Virologists recognize that a gap of at least 3-4 weeks is desirable between giving one vaccine and then a different one, because if not so spaced the immune response to the second vaccine may be inadequate and not produce sufficient specific antibodies to give protective immunity. If there is a dormant/latent viral infection already present in the recipient, vaccination against another pathogen could depress the immune system leading to the latent viral infection activating and expressing a new illness. This may be the case in cats, for example, who can come down with feline leukemia or herpes virus infections after receiving a feline distemper or rabies vaccine. Therefore, it concerns me that both humans, especially children, and animals are given combinations of vaccines—'cocktails'— all in one visit rather than carefully sequenced series of different vaccinations. It also concerns me that veterinarians seem to give little or no consideration to the role of vaccinations in the etiology of animal diseases, especially since more such cases are being widely diagnosed following repeat-vaccination of dogs and of certain canine breeds in particular.

In their discussion of possible causal co-factors in the genesis of neonatal pancytopenia in a herd of beef cattle, authors Bell and others (2010) make no mention of the potential role of vaccinations, the herd in question receiving six different booster vaccinations two months before the start of calving. Similarly, Shiel and others (2010) inexplicably did not raise the possibility of adverse vaccine reactions (vaccinosis) in a kennel of greyhounds all receiving several vaccinations prior to dogs developing nonsuppurative meningioencephalitis.

To make no mention of the possibility of vaccinosis may or may not reflect some taboo or complacent attitude toward questioning the role of modified live, attenuated and new-generation genetically engineered, DNA vaccines (and their adjuvant additives and substrate contaminants) in the aetiology of various disease conditions (Kamal 2009), notably those now increasingly diagnosed as auto-immune diseses (Duval & Giger 1996,Goggs and others 2008, Botch and others 2009).

Many modified live vaccines are grown on mammalian cells which can harbor retroviruses. Miyazawa and colleagues (2010) write: "The genomes of all animal species are colonized by endogenous retroviruses (ERVs). Although most ERVs have accumulated defects that render them incapable of replication, fully infectious ERVs have been identified in various mammals. In this study, we isolated a feline infectious ERV (RD-114) in a proportion of live attenuated vaccines for pets. Isolation of RD-114 was made in two independent laboratories using different detection strategies and using vaccines for both cats and dogs commercially available in Japan or the United Kingdom. This study shows that the methods currently employed to screen veterinary vaccines for retroviruses should be reevaluated."

Substrate contaminants have lead to adverse reactions such as kidney disease in cats (Lapin and others, 2006), and also to drug recalls, as with human measles vaccine contaminated with low levels of avian leukosis retrovirus, rotovirus vaccine with porcine circovirus, and Simian virus 40 in Polio vaccines possible leading to non-Hodgkin lymphoma (Vilchez et al 2002). Adjuvants added to vaccines to stimulate the immune response can also pose problems (Spickler & Roth 2003). Vaccines derived from cell cultures, such as from canine kidney cells, and intended for use in that same species, may cause auto-immune disease.

Veterinarians O'Toole and Van Campen (2010), expressing concern over the high incidence of abortions following cow vaccinations, particularly for bovine diarrhea virus, with MLV vaccines, for which there are over 150 different vaccination brands available, urge the government to require vaccine manufacturers to provide genetic sequence information to enable diagnosticians to be able to differentiate between vaccine and field strains of viruses causing animal health problems.

The correlation between vaccinations and neurological diseases in humans was demonstrated 15 years ago (Montinari and others 1996). Several human autoimmune diseases have been shown since then to be associated with both genetic factors and vaccinations (Orbach and others 2010). The latter authors state: "Infectious agents contribute to the environmental factors involved in the development of autoimmune diseases possibly through molecular mimicry mechanisms. Hence, it is feasible that vaccinations may also contribute to the mosaic of autoimmunity. Evidence for the association of vaccinations and the development of these diseases is presented in this review. Infrequently reported post-vaccination autoimmune diseases include systemic lupus erythematosus, rheumatoid arthritis, inflammatory myopathies, multiple sclerosis, Guillain-Barré syndrome, and vasculitis. In addition, we will discuss macrophagic myofasciitis, aluminum containing vaccines, and the recent evidence for autoimmunity following the use of human papillomavirus vaccine."

These two associations, i.e., genetics (breed) and vaccinations, in the aetiology of various diseases in dogs (Scott-Moncrieff and others, 2002), some hitherto believed to be of 'idiopathic' origin such as epilepsy and cutaneous atopy in dogs, have been reviewed (Dodds 2001, Hogenesch 1999); nutritional factors (Beck 2000) are also considerable, including prenatal and epigenetic influences. Adverse canine vaccination reactions were documented several years ago, notably interstitial nephritis and corneal opacity following vaccination with one type of infectious canine hepatitis (Appel and others 1973); encephalitis occurred when co-administered with a canine distemper virus vaccine (Cornwell and others 1988).

Vaccinoses—Adverse Vaccine Reactions

This is the roulette of vaccine-based preventive medicine. It has become an industry that we are learning to censor because of the increasing incidence of adverse vaccine reactions, so called vaccinosis, in human and companion animal recipients. Selling annual vaccinations along with manufactured, highly processed pet foods has become the bread and butter of conventional small animal veterinary practice. Yet this combination, like the consumer populace eating junk and convenience foods and being hypervaccinated in childhood, is the cause of a host of iatrogenic health problems, compounded by genetic susceptibility in certain pure-breeds and individuals.

Veterinarian W. J. Dodds (2001) has linked the following health problems in dogs to vaccinations that can harm some breeds more than others and appear more randomly in the 'mixed breed' segment of the population: Fever, stiffness, sore joints and abdominal tenderness, neurological disorders, polyneuropathy, transient seizures, and encephalitis, increased susceptibility to infections, collapse with autoimmune hemolytic anemia, immune mediated thrombocytopenia, immune-mediated hemolytic anemia, autoimmune thyroiditis, necrotizing vasculitis, joint disease, polyarthritis, and hypertrophic osteodystrophy. Hogenesch and others (1999) conducted several studies to determine if vaccines can cause changes in the immune system of dogs that might lead to life-threatening immune-mediated diseases such as lupus and glomerulonephrosis. The vaccinated, but not the nonvaccinated, dogs in the Purdue studies developed autoantibodies to many of their own biochemicals, including fibronectin, laminin, DNA, albumin, cytochrome C, transferrin, cardiolipin, and collagen. Autoantibodies to cardiolipin are frequently found in genetically susceptible patients with systemic lupus erythematosus, and also in individuals with other autoimmune diseases. The presence of elevated anti-cardiolipin antibodies is significantly associated with cardiomyopathy.

Vaccinosis prone dog breeds may mirror vaccinosis prone ethnic groups and individuals in the human population. Diabetes Types 1 & 2 have been linked to early vaccinations in human infants (Classen 1996). Montinari et al (1996) were the first to use immunogenetics to show the antigenic linkage between brain damage (demyelination) and a recombinant hepatitis vaccine in humans.

Interference or interreaction effects between different vaccines given in combination at the same time or separately at close intervals are a legitimate concern, potentially causing increased virulence and immunosuppression, or as Taguchi and others (2010) have shown, such immunization schedules depress the immune response and lower anitbody titers, which may prompt the expression of latent infection or autoimmune disease to arise.

Humans and other animals with inherited faulty B and/or T cell immunodeficiencies should not receive live-virus vaccines due to the risk of severe or fatal infection. B and T cell immunodeficiencies are also associated with food allergies, inhalant allergies, eczema, dermatitis, neurological deterioration, and heart disease.

Dog breeds vary in the titers they develop following vaccination, a low titer not necessarily meaning poor immunity, because of other components of immune defense mechanisms that blood titers do not measure, including mucosal immunity, cell-mediated immunity, and immune memory ells. The innate immune system modulates the quality and quantity of long-term T and B cell memory and protective immune response to pathogens.

Patients on steroidal and nonsteroidal anti-inflammatory drugs may not produce a good antibody response to vaccinations, while prior sensitization of dogs with an allergen such as pollen can lead to hypersensitivity associated with excess amounts of IgE antibodies and subsequent chronic inflammation of the skin, conjunctivitis and rhinitis.

Long-term over-activation of the immune system, as through

hyperimmunization with repeated annual 'booster' vaccinations, may be a major cause of cancer. Smith and Missailidis (2004) have proposed that inflammation could prevent the body from recognizing a foreign substance and may therefore serve as a hiding place for invaders. Cancers are like wounds that never heal and are surrounded by inflammation. This is generally thought to be the body's reaction to try to fight the cancer, but this may not the case. The inflammation is not the body trying to fight the infection. It is actually the virus or bacteria deliberately causing inflammation in order to hide from the immune system. That dogs surpass humans in the incidence of certain cancers raises the probability of hyperimmunization with MLVs which is a widespread practice in the US, the UK, Australia, and many other countries.

Holistic equine veterinarians have informed me that most horses are given so many different vaccines that many become immunocompromised. Vaccinating horses against West Nile virus can cause swelling in the front legs, fever, diarrhea and other systemic reactions like purpura hemorrhagica, urticaria and anaphylaxis. West Nile vaccine is also found to cause abortions in mares. Pickles and others (2011) found that 27 percent of horses given gonadotrophin-releasing hormone vaccinations had adverse reactions including one "severe, presumed immune-mediated myostitis" (Expressed as excruciating and potentially fatal muscular inflammation).

In part because of the immunocompromised condition of many racehorses infected with equine influenza, and who passed the infection on to greyhounds at the same track, a variant canine influenza vaccine is now marketed across the US.

The Behavior & Ecology of Viruses

Even seemingly harmless viruses like the coxsackievirus can become virulent in selenium-deficient human hosts (Beck,2000). Stress and malnutrition go hand in hand, impairing the immune system's ability to respond effectively against viral infections—and even against weaker strains in vaccines that then convey no immunity. Given this extreme variability of viruses that proliferate more as population densities increase, especially down on the CAFOs—confined and crowded animal feeding operations for pig, poultry and cattle industry 'farms,' we should not be adding to the genetic diversity of the viral community by introducing live GE vaccines. The same reservations hold true for the 'philanthropic' vaccination programs in the urban slums and impoverished rural communities where humans, rats, rabid dogs, and Ebola virus- and AIDS virus-carrying monkeys are part of the inter-species matrix for viral proliferation and evolution. We must look to safer and in the long term less costly solutions by addressing the ecology and behavior of infectious viruses.

The kinds of viral research going on today, including applications in biowarfare, are primarily driven to develop new vaccines to market in the name of 'preventive' human and veterinary medicine. The risks of genetically engineering new vaccines are considerable. We can pair the release of such GE vaccines into the environment with the recent reporting of the rabies virus rapidly evolving in Arizona and other parts of the US. It is cross-infecting bats, foxes, and skunks, and health authorities are rightly concerned that the virus could soon jump into the human population, like the Hanta virus and West Nile virus. Adding attenuated live vaccines into such a pathogenic milieu is counter-intuitive.

Using the proteins expressed from the rabies virus DNA, albeit replication-defective, and splicing it on to a highly attenuated avian influenza virus for manufacture and use by the poultry industry world wide, is patently absurd in terms of potential risks and ultimate costs. Widespread vaccinations against one infectious strain may open the door for the proliferation of a different pathogenic virus, as in the viral epidemic-vaccine associated outbreaks of canine distemper and rabies in Masai dogs, lions, wild dogs, and other endangered carnivore species. This is now being compounded by the spread of canine parvovirus into their communities.

The development of vaccines and biowarfare agents that can be dispensed as aerosols or nose-drops (in part justified in order to reduce adverse reactions to adjuvants in injected vaccines that can cause cancer and other diseases) has obvious military value. But such aerosol vaccines, like those of pig brains in mid-west slaughter houses that caused neurological disease in several workers, include foreign proteins that could trigger neurological and auto-immune diseases, allergic reactions and anaphylactic shock.

Safety & Consequences

Even if such government endorsed, pharmaceutical company funded, and 'philanthropically' supported institutions like the Jefferson Vaccine Center and Wistar Institute pass with flying colors on biosecurity, the actual biosafety of their new vaccines can only be really determined after they are released. The bioethics and biological consequences of these innovations have never been satisfactorily answered from a purely objective and scientific, rather than profit-driven, perspective. The same must be said with regard to the creation of vaccine-producing plants, like the potato with Hepatitis B oral vaccine that cooking will not destroy, and of genetically engineered and cloned farmed animals producing monoclonal antibodies in their milk and blood for use in 'the war on cancer' and other anthropogenic diseases. Developers of GE vaccines are gambling with life for primarily pecuniary ends, especially when the use of such vaccines is the primary if not sole response to potential pandemics and to the challenges of public health and disease prevention.

The misanthropy behind commercial vaccinology is more accident than design. Or so I wish to believe. The new generation of live GE vaccines being developed, tested and marketed could amount to a chaos-sustaining genetic pollution that will predictably be far worse than radioactive 'waste,' because it will be impossible to ever recall or contain. There are enough DNA-damaging pollutants in our food, water and air that need to be cleaned up as it is. Indirectly profiting from the health problems these are causing with ever more pharmaceutical and other conventional, often iatrogenic, medical treatments is ethically questionable. Infections to a large extent are anthropogenic, and so disease control has always been best achieved through such common sense applications of exposure risk, good hygiene, mechanical barriers/quarantine, and assuring good nutrition and healthy (especially noncrowded) environments.

It therefore may be prudent for those who are vaccinating billions of farmed and companion animals around the world to consider the long-term health and environmental implications of vaccines, and the related concerns being expressed and documented by virologists and other scientists over the safety, effectiveness and need for various vaccines currently being introduced into human and animal populations (Chan 2006, Traavik 1999). Because of the shorter lives of animals being killed for food, the long-term adverse effects of vaccinations may only be evident in longer-lived breeding stock. DNA vaccines that purportedly need no cold-chain preservation, are normally bacterial plasmids into which are spliced a promoter active in mammals, such as the cytomegalovirus promoter. This drives the coding sequence for an antigen. The plasmid is taken up by the mammalian cells and reaches the nucleus of some of those cells. There it is transcribed into RNA, which is translocated to the cytoplasm and translated into antigen protein. DNA vaccines thus induce a full spectrum of immune responses. These include antibodies, cytotoxic T lymphocytes, and T helper cells. Concerns have been expressed over the induction of autoimmunity and anti-DNA antibodies, which were observed in rabbits immunized with plasmids bearing a HIV reverse transcriptase gene.

Chan (2006), following up on the earler concerns expressed by T. Travik writes: "Despite major therapeutic advances, infectious diseases remain highly problematic. Recent advancements in technology in producing DNA-based vaccines, together with the growing knowledge of the immune system, have provided new insights into the identification of the epitopes needed to target the development of highly targeted vaccines. Genetically modified (GM) viruses and genetically engineered virus-vector vaccines possess significant unpredictability and a number of inherent harmful potential hazards. For all these vaccines, safety assessment concerning unintended and unwanted side effects with regard to targeted vaccinees has always been the main focus. Important questions concerning effects on nontargeted individuals within the same species or other species remain unknown. Horizontal transfer of genes, though lacking supportive experimental or epidemiological investigations, is well established. New hybrid virus progenies resulting from genetic recombination between genetically engineered vaccine viruses and their naturally occurring relatives may possess totally unpredictable characteristics with regard to host preferences and disease-causing potentials. Furthermore, when genetically modified or engineered virus particles break down in the environment, their nuclei acids are released. Appropriate risk management is the key to minimizing any potential risks to humans and environment resulting from the use of these GM vaccines. There is inadequate knowledge to define either the probability of unintended events or the consequences of genetic modifications."

Reliance on vaccinations as the cornerstone of preventive medicine and the top priority of the new 'One Health' movement being promoted by the BVA, AVMA, and World Health Organization among others, including philanthropic organizations such as the Bill & Melinda Gates Foundation and even some scientists in wildlife conservation and research, may be unwise, scientifically unsound, and medically unjustified when avoidable. Governmental health agencies' insistence on certain vaccinations, be they for children or animals, should recognize their full liablity to compensate victims for adverse reactions, and to empower attending physicians and veterinarians with the authority to grant waivers where there is informed consent or conditions where such blanket regulations are inappropriate, as with companion animals who are always kept indoors, farmed animals raised in accordance with organic farming standards, and all patients who are immunocompromised.

Above all, natural ecosystems must receive emergency CPR—conservation, preservation and restoration—analysis and action. Unhealthy, human-infested and degraded ecosystems are ideal environments for viruses to spill over from healthy carrier hosts, like bats who have brought us from their desecrated forests, the Hendra, Nipah and Ebola viruses that killed people and, respectively, horses, pigs and neighboring chimpanzees and gorillas. The Simian immuno-deficiency virus spilled over into humans as HIV-1. Anthropozootic diseases, which spread from people to wildlife, include polio, measles, influenza, and tuberculosis.

In the absence of relevant bioethics (Potter 1977 & Fox 2006), vaccinations and other medical and veterinary practices may cause more harm than good, especially when altruism is misguided and or uninformed, and the Earth's 'carrying capacity' and biodiversity-dependent functionality are not considered (Hardin 1977).

Vaccinations are neither the end-all of preventive medicine nor its proper foundation, but used with caution they may play a useful role in integrated (animal-human-environment) medicine and health care maintenance. The behavior of viruses would seem to make them an indicator bellweather species for us to monitor and understand for our own good rather than reflexively seek to eradicate them, since they reflect dysfunctional ecosystems and animal and human communities and populations.

Postscript: Vaccination Protocols for Companion Animals

The World Small Animal Veterinary Association (WSAVA) guidelines include the statement that "dogs that have responded to vaccination with MLV core vaccines (parvovirus, distemper virus and adenovirus) maintain immunity (immunological memory) for many years in the absence of any repeat vaccination." The 2007 WSAVA guidelines specifically warn that core vaccines should not be given any more frequently than every three years after the 12 month booster injection following the puppy/kitten series. The American animal Hospital Association's Canine Vaccine Task Force in 2003 noted that MLV vaccines are likely to provide lifelong immunity, stating "when MLV vaccines are used to immunize a dog, memory cells develop and likely persist for the life of the animal."

While the World Small Animal Veterinary Association now advocates a minimal 3-year interval between core 'booster' vaccinations for dogs and cats, the UK government's Veterinary Medicines Directorate (VMD) remains adamant that veterinarians should follow the manufacturers' guidelines posted on their website as per Pfizer Ltd Vanguard 7 Canine vaccine description in the VMDs Summary of Product Characteristics (SPC) (VMD.gov.uk/ProductinformationDatabase): "The duration of immunity for canine distemper virus, canine parvovirus, canine adenovirus type 1 and 2 and the leptospiral components are at least 12 months. However, the duration of immunity for canine parainfluenzavirus has not been determined. —Re-vaccination Scheme: A single dose of Vanguard 7 to be given annually thereafter" (Italics mine).

The VMD chief executive, Prof. Steve Dean, in a letter to the UK's Canine Health Concern, while acknowledging the WSAVA basic 3-year core vaccination regimen is accepted by many on clinical and science-based grounds, insists that the manufacturers' protocols published in the SPC, as per re-vaccination, should be adhered to by prescribing veterinarians, stating that "if departing from the SPC, veterinary surgeons do so under their own responsibility, and would be well advised to do so with the client's agreement."

Meeusen and others (2007) write: "A concern is that repeated vaccinations (with canarypox or other vectored vaccines) may result in immunity to the vector virus eliminating its ability to infect/transmit the desired genes to the immune system. Currently, several vectored vaccines are used in companion animals."

The U.S. Supreme Court ruling, Feb 22, 2011, to protect vaccine manufacturers from law suits following adverse reactions in children by denying parents the right to sue in state courts is a disturbing matter of public record. The US Congress set up an informal 'vaccine court' in 1986 to settle claims, paying out $1.9 billion to more than 2,500 plaintiffs. The case that went to the Supreme Court was rejected by the 'vaccine court' even though the child suffers from residual, post-vaccination seizures.

My thanks to W.Jean Dodds DVM, Patricia M. Jordan DVM & Scott Kale MD, JD, for input on this topic.For more detailed reviews of vaccination issues in animals, visit www.twobitdog.com/drfox/

"The only safe vaccine is one that is never used—No vaccine can be proven safe before it is given to children." Statements by the late James A. Shannon, while serving as Director of the US National Institutes of Health.

CHAPTER 15
Animal Welfare & Human Health:
Changing Ways in Medicine & Food

It is evident to most of us that there is a quickening of chaos all around, evoking a global angst embodied in the threats of terrorism, nuclear and bio-warfare, and catastrophic climate change and new pandemic diseases like the new human-avian-swine influenza virus. Is this part of the inevitable demise of *Homo technos*—anthropogenic nemesis? Or, are there solutions? In this chapter we will explore these issues, the dimensions of our pathology, and the horizons of survival and hope.

The end of living and the beginning of survival, as Chief Seattle once noted, is a reality today for millions of people, who are deprived of nutritious food, adequate clean water, and effective and affordable medicine. Their numbers are increasing world-wide as more people in the developed, industrialized world sink below the poverty line. The kind of main-stream, conventional Western medicine that is being practiced today, aside from emergency medicine, has become part of the disease-complex because of its iatrogenic (harmful, treatment-related) consequences.

Aggravated by the 'agricologenic' problems of food quality and safety, and people's poor food choices, the incidence of many diseases of Western civilization, such as cancer, metabolic, immunologic and psychiatric disorders, are increasing. The high incidence of bacterial food poisoning (1 in 4 persons annually, with 5,000 deaths and 300,000 hospitalizations according to the Centers for Disease Control), of obesity (1 in 5 children aged 4-years, and 1 in 3 if American Indian), and of diabetes (1 in every 3 children born after 2000 predicted to develop diabetes), indicate the urgent need for changing ways in medicine and food. Many similar diseases are evident in dogs and cats fed the byproducts of industrial agriculture processed into pet foods. Dogs have more cancers than humans (from www.caninecancer.com), and the leading cause of death from disease in children less than 14 years of age in the US is cancer.

Debates on health care reforms, government versus private health insurance schemes, and 'socialized medicine' will continue to be nothing more than hot air until everyone becomes enlightened about what they eat, how food is produced, and why food is no longer our first medicine for preventing disease.

Bad Medicine, Bad Food

The toxic agrichemical food industry, with its pesticides and genetically engineered, environmentally and health-hazardous crops, and the pharmaceutical industry with its farm animal vaccines and array of drugs given to inhumanely housed farmed animals, from antibiotics to steroids and adrenal stimulants, is capitalizing royally while putting the consumer populace at risk.

Atrazine, banned in many countries but the most widely used pesticide in the US, has been found in human amniotic fluid. It is an endocrine disruptor, feminizing male frogs; it is the most common contaminant in drinking water; and it may play a significant role in the obesity/metabolic syndrome.

Even genetically-engineered human growth hormone (known as rBST or rBGH) is injected into factory-farmed dairy cows in the US purely for profit as smaller dairy farms go our of business due to milk surpluses. This milk is altered, adulterated, and is considered by many health experts as unsafe; it may possibly increase the incidence of twin-births in the consumer-populace. In April 2009 a federal court in Ohio ruled that dairies cannot legally label their milk "hormone free" or "rBST-free" or otherwise clearly tell consumers that they are not pumping up their cows with synthetic hormones. This is a blow to truth-in-labeling advocates, a blow to consumers and a blow to organic farmers. It's a win for Monsanto, the agrichemical giant, and a win for Eli Lilly, which bought Monsanto's synthetic recombinant bovine growth hormone. The use of these hormones is banned throughout most other first world nations. Ohio was one of at least five states— including Pennsylvania, Missouri, Indiana and Kansas—where Monsanto launched quiet attacks on milk labeling through state agricultural departments.

The US government permits the release of other market products and services of such insanity as food irradiation, which are said to be 'safe' because they are 'regulated'. Food irradiation is rationalized as the ultimate solution to the bacterial contamination problem caused by crowding billions of poor creatures into confinement sheds and feedlots. These animals are fed inappropriate diets designed to force their growth and productivity, ignoring the fact that the environment within the gut allows for the proliferation of and shedding of pathogenic E. coli. The spread of E coli and salmonella in chickens is magnified through the processing of the animals after slaughter (See photo documentation at www.twobitdog. com/DrFox/). Researchers recently reported that cats fed irradiated food develop serous neurological problems and suffer extensive brain damage, such that many have to be euthanized. Residues of the ionophore Salinomycin in chickens, fed to stop a costly, management-created disease (coccidiosis), had very similar effects on cats eating contaminated poultry parts in their manufactured pet food.

Drug residues in animal products from the livestock, poultry and seafood industries add to the 'anthropogenic' nature of emerging diseases, from neuroendocrine dysfunctions to developmental and immune system disorders. Many of these emerging diseases of industrial society are associated clinically with hyperimmunization, and with adverse vaccine reactions in both human and animal recipients, especially in the over-vaccinated companion animal population that has a host of associated auto-immune and inflammatory diseases.

Profit-Driven 'Preventive' Medicine
Modified live and genetically engineered viruses used in vaccines, especially in livestock and poultry, and viruses like the Cauliflower mosaic virus used in virtually all genetically engineered crops, have the potential to mutate, recombine, and spread horizontally to nontarget species, insects being one group of potential vectors. We have seen how the swine flu virus has mutated to infect poultry, then cats and dogs, and then humans. Some virologists fear further mutation and combination with HIV and Hepatitis B viruses.

Cancer is primarily a disease of immune system breakdown. Both vaccine adjuvants (like carcinogenic aluminum salts, and mutagenic and immunosuppressive mercury thimerasol) and antigenic proteins in the modified live and genetically engineered (GE) vaccines, may precipitate a cancerous event in recipients, along with a host of complex auto-immune diseases. It is a tragic irony that man's best friend, the dog, has a higher rate of cancer of the skin, breast, bone, and lymph system (leukemia) than his caretaker. This immune-and gene-dysfunction syndrome is the dog's primary cause of death, after 'old age', according to two recent Scandinavian veterinary surveys.

The health consequences of routine 'preventive' use of many new broad-spectrum anti-parasite and flea drugs in dogs and cats, and their environmental impact, give much cause for concern. The Environmental Protection agency received over 44,000 reports of adverse reactions to topical anti-flea and tick drugs in cats and dogs in 2008. Similar drugs are used widely by the livestock industry. Without concurrent exposure to a host of other food and environmental toxins, such products might be a little less of a concern for companion animal health (See Polluted Pets, by the Environmental Working Group, 2008, that shows high levels of industrial chemicals contaminating dogs and cats).

The new paradigm of the 'one medicine'—human and animal— is the antithesis of conventional, primarily interventive, medicine. Conventional human and veterinary medicine is also over-capitalized (especially in diagnostic services rather than preventive), and promotes vaccinations as preventive medicine while not addressing the *causes* of disease. Most highly contagious diseases are pluricausal and multifactor and are not simply a consequence of high virulence and contagiousness; one example is the Ebola virus recently discovered in Philippine pig farms, and in humans working and living in pig farming communities. Most microorganisms are not harmful pathogens until they have the right host environment in which to proliferate, and a factory pig farm is one such ideal environment.

The new strain of swine flu, A/H1N1 includes genetic material from swine, poultry and human variants, and underscores the contribution of high densities of farmed animals serving as Petri-dishes for the evolution of zoonotic diseases, which are compounded by human proximity, international travel, and trade, especially in live animals. The US government will spend $2 billion of public funds in contracting drug companies to fast-track vaccine production to combat this new influenza strain, a policy decision based on fear and ignorance, if not also pandering to corporate interests regardless of the potential risks, questionable need and effectiveness of such a vaccine. Vaccinations will be given without adequate testing for safety and effectiveness, and the Government has ruled that manufacturers are immune from law suits over adverse reactions.

Emerging disease like Lyme's and West Nile disease, avian influenza, and MRSA (methicillin-resistant staphylococcus aureus) can best be prevented by appropriate environmental health management policies and humane farming practices, rather than with new vaccines and drugs that the pro-agricultural biotechnology/GM crop-advocating Rockefeller Foundation, in its One Health Commission (JAVMA, 234:p992, 2009), is helping promote. Some 75 percent of emerging diseases over the past 30 years involve the veterinary profession since they are zoonotic (animal-to-human transmitted). More appropriate and effective management policies and programs would not rely on drugs and vaccinations, but on providing more humane and healthful environments for farmed animals, and proper wildlife management through ecosystem CPR (conservation, preservation, and restoration) rather than trap- and -poison methods of predator and pest control.

Looking to the Future

As economies, ecologies and cultures continue to collapse around us, we can all find ways to wellness, through living simply, mindfully, and supporting local and organic food producers and markets; and by becoming 'kitchen anarchists,' preparing our own meals with known ingredients from known sources, and those for our animal companions as well. Our food should be our first medicine. Imported soy products from China bearing the USDA label of Organic Certification may not be up to US producer standards and can be contaminated with hexane, a chemical used in processing that is an environmental pollutant and neurotoxin. Diet drinks laced with US government approved aspartame is another source of neurotoxin, while the herbal sweetener, Stevia, though more costly, may actually help lower blood sugar and reduce insulin tolerance.

The economic and environmental— especially climate change— problems that future generations will face could be greatly ameliorated today by a massive reduction in the global cattle population, from Colorado and Iowa to India and Australia. For public health reasons alone the globally expanding pig and poultry populations, greatly encouraged by the World Bank, must be cut back and replaced with humane, organic, and sustainable production methods as were practiced before global colonization by the 'agribusiness' food industry. And we should all eat lower on the food chain for both health and environmental reasons.

That the Amazon jungle and indigenous peoples, and the last of Indonesia's rain forests and the Sumatran tiger are facing annihilation by the logging industry and soy and palm oil plantations respectively, is a travesty, and part of the profit-driven insanity of these increasingly dysfunctional times. (Palm oil, like soy oil, is high in pro-inflammatory omega 6 fatty acids, both being used in the West by the food industry, and palm cake and soy meal are used in farmed animal feed and poor quality pet foods). To continue on their present course, the hegemony of the multinational corporations will mean the impoverishment of future generations, and the war between the rich and poor, the greedy and the needy, will intensify.

The Food and Drug Industry Alliance

The Food and Drug Industry Alliance (FDIA, my acronym), a shadowy unofficial linkage of the major multinational oligopolies of agriculture, food and petrochemical-pharmaceutical industries tries to regulate itself in the US under the paid-for-by-the-public federal Food and Drug Administration (FDA). The FDIA donates millions of dollars to professional organizations like the American Medical Association and the American Veterinary Medical Association, as well as to human and veterinary medical colleges. Rather than advocating humane alternatives to raising animals under the pathogenic environments of confinement feeding operations, organized human and veterinary medicine have given the animal agriculture industry a free hand with a host of drugs, toxic chemicals and live virus vaccines for far too long.

Simply advising people to 'eat more whole grains, fruits and vegetables' is not an appropriate or adequate medical response by Government to the current consumer-health crisis. The pharmaceutical industry would oppose any reductions in farmed animal numbers since their mission is market expansion—now into developing countries under the missionary zeal of US Embassies and Consular offices around the world—just as they have effectively blocked any restrictions on the nontherapeutic use of antibiotics and other drugs used to boost the productivity of factory farmed animals. So would the agribusiness petrochemical fertilizer and pesticide manufacturers and commodity crop industries, like those of cotton, corn and soy (now predominantly genetically modified/GM) that market human processed foods, farmed animal feed, and manufactured pet foods also oppose reductions in numbers. (Cotton oil and cake is used in many processed foods and as byproducts in farmed animal feed. Sheep in India have been killed by toxins in GM cotton). The Cattlemen's Association and the National Pork Producers, along with the ranchers and other abusers of Public Lands, join those who see climate change as something to deny rather than properly address, and refuse to acknowledge their contribution to this serious issue.

The Obama administration's approval of GM sugar beet in April 2009 shows the power of the FDIA—This is an ominous ruling that should be reversed. The US Dept. of Agriculture rubber stamped the release of GM sugar beets without preparing an environmental impact statement, which is required by the National Environmental Policy Act. Obama chose Tom Vilsack, former Governor of Iowa and a long-time supporter of agricultural biotechnology, as USDA Secretary. Vilsack uses the emotional blackmail of the FDIA, which calls any opposition to GM crops as being anti-humanitarian.

The food and drug industry alliance's claim that theirs is the best and only way to feed a hungry world that cannot farm without pesticides, chemical fertilizers, genetically engineered seeds and hybrid and cloned farmed animals is patently absurd, and has no scientific validity. Research has shown that organic farming methods, especially in developing countries, can be three times more productive than most current farming practices, and can be as productive when input costs are considered, than the predominant industrial farming systems of Western agribusiness (referenced in *Nature* 2000). They are also more sustainable, soil-enriching and energy-conserving; and also climate-stabilizing (according to George Monbiot, *The Guardian*, 2000, among many).

Misguided Philanthropy?

Bill Gates is giving billions of dollars to encourage African and other poor nation states to accept GM crops, and to support mass infant vaccinations and canine anti-rabies vaccinations—but all to what end? It is no coincidence that he holds strategic investments in both agribiotechnology and the drug industry, whose products his nonprofit foundation strongly lobbies for.

Without being integrated with family planning, and local self-sufficiency, from clean water to fertile soil, the human population will continue to suffer and spread like a cancer on the Earth. Malnutrition in children and animals can reduce the effectiveness of vaccinations, increase the probability of adverse reactions, and increase the virulence of even normally harmless virus strains like the Coxsackie virus. Humane population control in dogs (through spay/neuter), coupled with vaccinations and humane education that includes proper nutrition, have been shown to be the best ways to keep rabies out of third-world communities because vaccinations alone are as ineffectual as traditional mass killings as practiced in China and India.

Human-focused altruism will be our species' nemesis. The road to hell is clearly paved with good intentions. Or is such vaccine and super-GM seed promotion a feel-good, 'win-win' delusion of the ill informed? Surely it is not simply to sell more products in a highly competitive and increasingly dysfunctional world market that such vested interests helped create in the first place. That is not a good investment even in the short term for those who put their faith and trust in the science and promises of the food and drug industrial complex. I agree with Jonathan Porritt who reasons, in his book *Capitalism as if the World Matters* (Earthscan Pub.

Ltd., 2005), that the current political primacy of key social goals, such as the elimination of poverty or the attainment of universal human rights, should become secondary to the biological imperative to learn to live sustainably on this planet, and cause less harm. He calls this "an absolute imperative, in that it is determined by the laws of nature and, hence, is non-negotiable—"

Making a Difference

Those fortunate to have any choice in this market place can help make a difference in many ways for their own good and for the ultimate good of the planet. There is no reason why the FDA or FDIA cannot do the same.

To take care means to take charge of our own health and that of our loved ones. This includes our companion animals, as well as those animals on our farms and in the wild. Health advocacy must include environmental advocacy, with healthy forests and wildlife meaning less global warming and more clean air and water. It must also include sustainable farming methods that do not poison surface and ground waters, and that enrich the soil and therefore the food we eat, so that our food is indeed our first medicine.

The anarchism of taking charge means taking personal responsibility for our health and for those for whom we care—for 'all our relations' as traditional Native American Indians proclaim. To them this is 'good medicine', and it includes respect for the environment and all living things. What we call Nature they call the Medicine Wheel. The Wheel is broken and they have become obese, depressed and diabetic. In the dominant world view of secular materialism this 'break' calls for sound science and economics, and rigorous global, rather than simplistic medical bioethics, which is empathy-based and fosters eco-justice as well as social justice, and compassion toward all sentient life.

So-called philanthropists fund nonprofit organizations to help promote expensive and hazardous pharmaceutical products and GM crops to ostensibly heal and feed the hungry world, and at the same time is investing in these industries rather than in more holistic, integrative, and sustainable approaches to human health and welfare (For insights go to http://www4.dr-rath-foundation.org/THE_FOUNDATION/microsoft.htm). I find this behaviour of the rich and powerful, unconscionable, perversely misanthropic, and morally inverted by some distorted faith in science and technology.

I find hope in the emerging practices of integrative, holistic preventive medicine and treatment protocols for animals as well as for humans. As Hippocrates advised, "Let our food be our medicine, and our medicine be our food." Organic farming practices are part of good medicine, vital to public health, since several studies have confirmed the higher nutritional value of organically produced foods because organic soils are richer in micronutrients than chemically fertilized soils producing commodity monocultures with no crop rotation or fallowing of the land. The medical health benefits of herbs and nutraceuticals are also being confirmed and marketed, as physicians and veterinarians acknowledge the risks of hyperimmunization and of over-prescribing antibiotics, corticosteroids and many other drugs that harm more than they help through misuse. Many widely prescribed pharmaceuticals are now being detected in our drinking water and in the rain; even antibiotics fed to livestock and poultry are being detected in crops fertilized with the farmed animals' manure.

The new healing paradigm of pyschoneuroimmunoenhancement is being practiced by more and more medical and veterinary doctors and by alternative and indigenous healers. A disillusioned and sickening populace is turning to such health care providers as the conventional, drug-and vaccine dependent, iatrogenic medical industry and its insurance and drug company oligopolies founder along with the 'global' economy. The industry responds by trying to outlaw the nonprescription sales of many tried and true alternative herbal, nutraceutical and other health care products.

The spiritual well-being of patients has been a neglected element of both veterinary and human medicine for decades. This is now changing as caregivers recognize: The significance of the patents' emotional state and will to live; the harms of 'hospitalism's' dissociative and depressive states; the importance of appropriate human contact including massage and physical/behavioral therapy; and for animal as well as human patients, an environment that provides comfort, security and freedom from fear. The institutionalized stupefaction of nursing home and other patients with psychotropic drugs should become a thing of the past. Parents are questioning the use of similar drugs in their children for attention-deficit and hyperactivity problems that good nutrition can do much to prevent, along with better emotional care and understanding. The same is true for companion animals in whom the use of psychotropic drugs for various behavioral problems has been promoted by the pharmaceutical industry, but thanks to many caring veterinarians, the exclusion of effective dietary considerations and nondrug behavioral therapies is generally avoided.

The psychological problems, alcoholism, family violence, and crime in disintegrating indigenous communities call for more than new medicines, vaccines and law enforcement. Unless, that is, there is no real intent to find any solution to over-population and instead simply sell false hope and reap great profits while the process of cultural euthanasia continues. But the forces of nature, from desertification to mass plagues and pestilence, will intensify if there is no effective family planning that some regard as genocidal, and if equal priority is not given to planetary CPR—conservation, preservation, and restoration of natural ecosystems. Otherwise the triage zones of human despair, from one landless refugee camp to another, will expand across the globe, threatening far more than 'national security.'

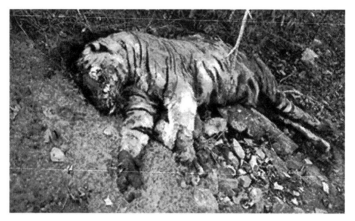

Figure 15-1. Tiger poisoned in Nilgiri, South India (M.W. Fox)

An Ethic of Care

The Hippocratic Oath 'Do no harm' applies not only to physicians but to consumers, producers, manufacturers, governments, and corporations. There is enough uncertainty and chaos in an emergent cosmos where cataclysmic and apocalyptic forces are at work, and about which we need more understanding and preparation, without our adding further chaos of an anthropogenic nature. In the final analysis an ethic of care is the second and maybe the best medicine—Food is the first medicine—for a sickening and increasingly dysfunctional planet. It is the basis for a sane society, a viable economy, and a healthy environment for all. The bioethical connections between human health and well-being, environmental conservation, restoration and preservation, and animal welfare and rights, must be incorporated into all realms of government, public policy and action, as well as the law.

CHAPTER 16
Wildlife Conservation, Animal Protection
& Human Wellbeing: An Essential Unity

Synopsis
International efforts to improve human health and wellbeing are now recognizing that such efforts will not succeed if the quality of the human environment is ignored. Improving environmental quality is an integral component of 'planetary CPR' —environmental conservation, preservation, and restoration.

The importance of improving the health and welfare of domestic animals as an integral component of both 'planetary CPR' and improving human health and wellbeing, is now also gaining recognition. For too long, animal welfare and protection have taken a low priority on the philanthropic, international aid, development, and humanitarian agenda. This overview of the essential connections between people, animals and nature presents the case for a more integrative approach to wildlife conservation, human wellbeing, and domestic animal protection and health.

Re-visioning Health
The old definition of health as the absence of disease has been broadened by the World Health Organization to include social, economic and environmental considerations. This broader definition may be adequate for urban people, especially those of the industrial West. But for the majority of the world's rural communities and indigenous (tribal) peoples, it is insufficient. It is inadequate for the formulation of appropriate policies and implementation of effective aid and development programs, because the health and welfare of the domestic animals living with these people and the protection of wildlife, conservation and restoration of natural habitat ('biodiversity' and 'ecosystems') are integral to human wellbeing, on many levels. These include public health, family nutrition, economic security, community sustainability, cultural identity, and traditional and spiritual values. Biodiversity and cultural diversity are interlinked, codependent and co-evolved in all ecosystems that include the human species

Global Biosphere Reserves

The brilliance of the United Nations Man and the Biosphere initiative, which has now identified over 400 Global Biosphere Reserves around the world, is in the recognition of this vital linkage between culture and Nature, and between the integrity of cultural and biological diversity. Integrity does not imply a preservationist paradigm that seeks to freeze the human and wild and domestic animal and plant co-communities in some kind of static limbo in time and space. Such limbos would be virtual realities, akin to theme parks, requiring constant and costly external correctives.

The Biosphere II project, the experimental, hi-tech but closed human, plant and animal biotic community in the Arizona desert, failed to be a self-regenerative biosystem because of unforeseen consequences that led to a decreasing supply of oxygen. A sustainable, low-input, regenerative biosphere system is one that is open, fluid, and biodynamic, rather than closed, controlled, and 'biostatic.'

Sustainable Biosystems

Sustainable human biosystems are the antithesis of the agricultural, agroforestry and aquatic monocultures of the industrial age. Self-sustaining systems incorporate and enhance biodiversity through locally and bioregionally appropriate polycultures of various domestic plants and animals (i.e. mixed farming, forestry and aquaculture systems); and through the sustainable management and exploitation of natural resources, including wild animals from bees to buffalo, who are treated humanely because they are respected as integral to the wellbeing of both the human community and the entire biotic community.

The factors that are endangering both indigenous peoples and wildlife—biocultural diversity—in many of these UN-designated Global Biosphere Reserves often have a synergistic effect, as I discovered and documented in one of these Reserves in Southern India. The Honey Kurumba tribals in this Nilgiri Biosphere Reserve in Tamil Nadu traditionally adopt sustainable use and management practices of forest resources, including the wax and honey of wild bees, which are now endangered, along with the Kurumbas and other tribal peoples. The Toda tribal pastoralists in this same Reserve, for example, face illegal land encroachment of the traditional grazing lands and the near extinction of their unique Toda white buffalo that are integral to their cultural identity and religion, from a lack of adequate veterinary services. (See details below.)

I worked with my wife Deanna Krantz in India for several years where her project advocated and activated several integrated programs based on an expanded World Health Organization (WHO-UN) vision of health and human wellbeing. This expanded vision linked the health and wellbeing of domestic animals, upon whom the indigenous peoples are dependent, economically, culturally, and spiritually, with the health and conservation of wildlife.

The protection of wildlife, conservation and restoration of natural habitat, are linked with the traditional and innovative sustainable farming methods and other community-based, environmentally friendly activities, including social forestry and soil and water conservation practices of indigenous peoples.

The Animal Component

This holistic, integrated paradigm means that this equation holds:

Healthcare = Peoplecare + Animalcare + Earthcare.

A healthy domestic animal population—achieved through free community veterinary services, humane education, training in animal husbandry, and enforcement of animal anti-cruelty laws—means improved income for livestock keepers, and control of zoonotic diseases (like rabies and foot and mouth disease) that unhealthy domestic animal populations harbor and variously spread to people and wildlife.

We put into practice a working model project whose replication in other Global Biosphere Reserves would do much to ensure the continued protection and restoration of biocultural diversity because of its grass-roots, rather than top-down, approach of working with the people for the people. Animal welfare is to human welfare, as nature conservation and biodiversity are to human culture and diversity. Hence, the value of an interdisciplinary approach where improvement in the human condition is linked with improving environmental quality, wildlife and habitat conservation, preservation, and restoration, and with domestic animal health, productivity, and welfare through improved veterinary care and humane husbandry education.

More recent, post-colonial efforts to protect wildlife and habitat have involved indigenous peoples in such roles as working as wildlife eco-safari trackers, conservation monitors, and anti-poaching teams; in reducing the adverse impacts of their domestic animals through improved grazing, land management practices, and animal health and productivity; and by adopting economically viable, sustainable agricultural practices and cooperative, socially just marketing networks.

Similar kinds of illegal and legal activities, from poaching and diverting streams to grazing too many animals and poisoning and snaring predators, as we documented in the Nilgiri Biosphere Reserve (see Addendum), are likely to be encountered in other Global Biosphere Reserves. Hence, the need for close collaboration with reliable local NGOs, government officials, village leaders, and tribal elders who understand the need for reform, collaborative oversight and effective management, coupled with appropriate animal protection and conservation law enactment and consistent enforcement, and the implementation of economically viable, environmentally friendly, and socially just ways to meet the needs of the people.

International organizations like Wildlife Conservation International, and Heifer Project International are adopting the bottom-up rather than top-down approach, working with local NGOs and government authorities at the grass roots, putting compassion into action, and facilitating mutually enhancing symbioses between people, animals, and Nature.

The critical state of the world's ecosystems and precarious future of most indigenous communities present a global triage situation for those governmental and nongovernmental organizations dedicated to human aid and development, and to saving the last of the wild. The UN Global Biosphere Reserve initiative identifies those places and peoples that, given the finite nature of financial and other external inputs and resources, have the best chance of being conserved, protected, and restored.

Wildlife Research Needs Ethical Boundaries & Veterinary Supervision

There are several documented, and many word-of mouth accounts of chemically immobilized and otherwise restrained endangered species like the Asian elephant and African wild dog being severely injured, killed or dying soon after capture and/or release. In some instances there was an association with the animals being injected with untested and unapproved modified live virus vaccines. In other instances the injured or killed animal was a pregnant or nursing mother.

Experienced veterinary supervision is called for especially when research biologists are loose in the field using drugs and vaccines on their animal subjects and applying various methods of capture and restraint which may cause serious injury, capture myopathy and even death.

Wildlife continue to be harassed, stressed, and subjected to these in-field risks so that tissue and blood samples can be taken (though DNA evidence can be obtained from feces and rubbing/marking areas), radio collars and cameras fitted, and microchips implanted. The generation of more scientific data from such field research may help advance careers and engender more funding, and give some substance to wildlife management schemes. But when the animals in question are put at risk, and there are no in-place regulations and effective law enforcement to protect and restore their existing habitats, and to extend the same in order to help minimize accelerating loss of genetic biodiversity, then these wildlife researchers should cease and desist.

Such activities alone have nothing to do with wildlife conservation and at best give the false impression that something is being done, or that the foreign presence alone is a deterrent to poaching and destruction. Yet in reality, from a bioethical perspective, the risks to the animals far exceed the immediate and foreseeable benefits. So I appeal to all appropriate institutions, governmental and nongovernmental, for-profit and not-for profit, to encourage alternative, noninvasive wildlife research, and to cease funding and permitting any form of wildlife capture except for urgent veterinary and conservation-translocation reasons.

A Case Study: Problems in the Nilgiri Global Biosphere Reserve
Thanks to an information network of villagers and tribal peoples who had intimate knowledge of the jungle, and who came to trust our in-field CPR (conservation, preservation and restoration) work in the Nilgiris that began in 1995, we were able to document and report to the appropriate authorities various illegal activities in the Global Biosphere Reserve, which the local people could not do for fear of reprisal, even death.

These illegal activities invaded every sector and included:
• Construction of guest lodges, tea shops and temples;
• The operation of a brick factory in restricted areas;
• Land encroachment for agriculture;
• Grazing livestock in restricted areas;
• Illegal diversion of rivers and streams into private lands and pumping water from the same to irrigate cash-crops, and pollution of same by agrichemicals and small industries;
• Expansion of eucalyptus, tea and coffee plantations that seriously depleted and variously polluted the water table;
• Opening up of new roads and illegal improvement of forest roads in the Reserve restricted for use by Forest and Wildlife Departments only;
• Illegal cutting of trees for firewood and lumber;

- Nonsustainable, destructive harvesting of forest products (mosses, lichens, gooseberries, soap nut, tamarind, etc.);
- Movement of unquarantined, uninspected and infected livestock into the Reserve;
- Sport hunting, poaching, and sale of wild meat, skins, elephant ivory and other wildlife products;
- Killing elephants and other wildlife with homemade bombs and by shooting, electrocuting, poisoning, and snaring ('snoosing');
- Illegal removal of cattle manure and the quarrying and removal of rocks and sand;
- Burning of the remains of killed elephants and endangered wildlife guar, tiger, leopard by forest staff to avoid punishment for not catching the killers;
- Procurement of tribal girls for prostitution at local guest lodges, and the killing and suicides of same;
- Misappropriation of foreign funds, which were provided to empower tribal women and to facilitate family planning and economic security, but were used to bribe officials, purchase land and vehicles and to build a guest lodge for eco-tourism;
- Illegal receipt and misappropriation of foreign donations and government funds to operate a bogus animal shelter and refuge that provided no free services to the local community as mandated by its Charter of Incorporation;
- Bribing of various government employees, including high-ranking government officials, roadside check-post officers, police and SPCA animal welfare inspectors, veterinarians falsifying livestock numbers, vaccination records and autopsy reports on wild and domestic animals;
- And, providers and purchasers of contaminated and inferior grade food for captive elephants falsifying receipts, and elephant caretakers falsifying body weight, injury and treatment records.

The Indian Institute of Science (IIS) enabled a German student to bring several hives of domesticated bees into the Nilgiri Reserve to study their behavior and adaptability, an extremely irresponsible project that could endanger the wild bees through contagious infections and competition, and thus endanger the traditional sustainable economy of the Honey Kurumbas. IIS scientists have been doing research studies on elephants and other wildlife for decades in the Nilgiris, accidentally killing some, for instance, by tranquilizing elephants for radio-collaring. They have shown no evidence of any active and effective involvement in species and habitat protection and restoration at the local level, where it is clearly needed and involves cooperative efforts with local peoples and government officials. Doing research for its own sake, and not getting involved in the politics of CPR, as elephants and other endangered species are on the brink of extinction, is irresponsible, like Nero fiddling while Rome burns.

Other government and nongovernment projects like tree planting, introduction of 'improved' water buffalo, and growing feed and fodder for local livestock have failed over the years due to poor management, lack of oversight, misappropriation of funds, and limited if any consultation with village leaders and tribal elders, whose wisdom is rarely appreciated.

Other major problems included increasing human incursion and settlement with increased pressure on water and fuel wood resources; the accidental introduction of a highly invasive weed like Stephasegria in imported crop seeds; the abandonment of growing traditional, rain-fed and highly nutritious varieties of staple crops like ragi for local consumption; and, a high population of 'scrub' cattle raised primarily as manure producers (for out-of-state sale as organic fertilizer) and which are extensively grazed, become extremely malnourished. These cattle suffer terribly during the dry season, compete with wildlife, and spread disease.

CHAPTER 17
The 'Greening' of Animal & Human Medicine
Revisioning Disease: Nature-Nurture Co-Factors

To enter modern civilization is indeed to enter disease. To advocate alternative, complementary treatments integrated with the conventional is to challenge the political and economic status quo as well as a limited, corporate-profit-driven medical paradigm. It is limited because of a lack of any integrated approach to treatment of disease and prevention. Instead, it tends to rely on intervention and more recently on addressing genetic/genomic co-factors to the exclusion of environmental co-factors.

The co-factors underlying many infectious and noninfectious diseases, and their prevention, are genetic and endogenous; environmental and exogenous: nature and nurture. Expensive drugs, often with harmful side-effects, DNA screening, and recombinant DNA vaccines to influence genetic co-factors, are now a top research and development priority for the medical industry. This is in part because of increasing bacterial resistance to antibiotics resulting from their misuse by the livestock and poultry industries, and resistance to making long-overdue improvements in how farmed animals are husbanded. In the U.S., according to the Union of Concerned Scientists, 16 percent of antibiotics are used to treat humans and companion animals, while 14 percent is used to treat sick farm animals, and 70 percent is put in their feed to enhance productivity. Genetic resistance to pesticides in crop and animal pests and parasites due to the indiscriminate and wholesale use of these chemicals is all part of the same food and agriculture originating, environmental co-factor sector of many animal and human diseases.

Expensive anti-viral, gene-targeting, genome-altering drugs, genetically engineered live vaccines, and gene-slicing and silencing biotechnologies are being researched and developed for both the medical and agribusiness food industries to better combat human, animal, and plant diseases.

The iatrogenic (treatment-induced) consequences of earlier kinds of vaccines and the adjuvants and other additives and contaminants therein continue to be dismissed by organized medicine, a problem that pales in my mind before the veterinary profession's unquestioned support of stressful, inhumane and disease-promoting intensive methods of animal production from their inception, and continued foot-dragging over their food animal sector role and responsibilities in the very serious issue of antibiotic resistance.

Public concerns were swept aside in the rapid U.S. government approval of anabolic steroids, systemic pesticides, genetically engineered bovine growth hormone and other Big Pharm 'animal health and productivity' pharmaceuticals, many of which are banned in other countries for consumer health, environmental and animal welfare concerns.

Human-Caused Diseases

The iatrogenic consequences of antibiotics and chemical pesticides, compounded by chemical fertilizers, nutrient-deficient soils, forages and crops, and by how the land is farmed and animals raised, promote disease. These environmental co-factors play an instrumental role in the genesis of new kinds of often virulent infections, and sometimes highly contagious viral, mycobacterial, protozoal, fungal and other diseases. Noninfectious metabolic, neuro-endocrine, immunologic, developmental, and reproductive disorders are linked to these and other environmental and genetic co-factors. Those genetic co-factors (including genetic uniformity/lack of biodiversity) in hybrid varieties of crops and farmed animals selected for high yield traits, and the selective breeding of pure-bred dogs, cats, and other domestic animals for extreme, biologically anomalous physical characteristics, are recognized by many as pervasive but not insurmountable concerns.

Chemical and pharmacological residues in what we consume, as well in our companion animals, are known carcinogens and endocrine-disruptors. These, along with the nutrient deficiencies, questionable additives and adulterants in many manufactured and processed foods and beverages, are some of the co-factors involved in the genesis of many noninfectious diseases, especially obesity, diabetes, cancer, heart disease, and allergies. They also play a significant role in lowering resistance to infectious diseases. Nutritionists are at last reaching unanimity over one major disease co-factor, namely omega fatty acid deficiencies and imbalances in the foods that we and our animal companions consume, and in the fats and oils in which many foods are cooked.

Neglected Environment & Disease Co-Factors

There is little profit incentive for the multinational food and drug industrial complex and allied medical and animal health industries to address the environmental/exogenous co-factors of infectious and noninfectious diseases. Aside from the epigenetic effects of some environmental co-factors, many of these co-factors we share with our companion animals because of where and how we live, and what we all ingest. According to Veterinary Pet Health Insurance, the conditions most often reported in insurance claims in the U.S. in 2008, which are common to both human and animal patients (but not transmissible from one species to the other) were, in descending order of prevalence: Allergies, bladder infection, arthritis, diabetes, skin cancer, and gum disease.

Today's house cats and home dogs are the canaries down the proverbial mine shaft, which they share with us. Environmental co-factors could be addressed at far less cost and risk than some of the more interventive treatments currently being advocated, such as using genetic engineering to enhance disease resistance, prescribing DNA vaccines, and costly and often harmful immunosuppressive chemotherapies, radiation, and immune-system enhancing drugs. Most often the symptoms of disease and inflammation are treated repeatedly with conventional, less costly drugs such as antibiotics and corticosteroids, with harmful side-effects.

Environmental co-factors in food animal production, such as over-crowding stress, poor sanitation, ventilation and building design, and body injuries and death in transit to slaughter are written off as one of the inevitable costs of high-volume production, the so-called economy of scale. This 'bigger the better' business model spawned ever larger and more intensely crowded animal factory farms and feedlots that are now epicenters for zoonotic diseases, environmental pollution, and water and food contamination—they are also places of unspeakable animal suffering, which I first documented some thirty years ago, along with the puppy breeding mills, on many once viable family farms.

Economies of scale and pure greed notwithstanding, the global economic crisis of 2010 was caused in part by corporate entities becoming "too big to fail." The increasing complexity of any corporate enterprise can quickly become dysfunctional, just like the health care system with its layers of insurance-dictated treatments, legal administrative costs, and federal regulations, while drug companies continue to raise prescription drug prices and, with the support of politicians, seek periodically to ban all OTC (over-the-counter) nonprescription products such as vitamins and other nutraceutical supplements. Many tried and true home remedies, traditional wisdom, and even common sense personal health care maintenance habits and customs, are going the way of the trusting Dodo bird.

A Clearer Vision
We need a medical paradigm of such scope that profits do not exclude compassion, and scientific 'proof' does not trump evidence-based medicine. We need health education that empowers consumer awareness, a health and environmentally conscious consumerism promoted by government, along with the Green anarchy of the humane and conscientious cook and kitchen.

We need a vision of health based on the principles of symbiogenetic balance, harmony and dynamic instability as well as full attention to the above disease co-factors rather than that of the medical Imperium with its 'war' on cancer and 'battle' against birth defects. We need a medicine and health care system for humans and other animals based more on well-being and disease prevention than on interventive treatments when diseases occur.

We need a medical vision of health that sees the culture-crippled and de-humanizing distortions of the human condition getting ever worse, as long as those cultural values, perceptions and beliefs are adhered to that lead to so much intra-species violence (internecine strife), animal cruelty and suffering, extinction of wildlife, and violence against the natural world.

This is the 'Greening' of the human and animal health care industries, which I did not expect to live to see, but is happening now, as witnessed by one multinational pet food manufacturer marketing its own brand of beneficial dietary probiotics for cats and dogs; the plethora of many good quality pet foods and nutraceutical supplements in the market place; increasing consumer demand for organically certified foods. More and more human and animal doctors are moving away from conventional treatment protocols and are adopting a balanced approach which gives due attention to all disease co-factors and integrates complementary and alternative treatments to health problems that can be rectified with the least harm or risk to the patient.

The prescribing of veterinary and human drugs that remain active in the environment after being excreted by the recipients and contaminate our drinking water, our food, and even the rain, and harm wildlife and ecosystems, is a concern high on the agenda of 'Green' medicine. This issue of pharmaceutical eco-toxicosis is a serious exogenous disease co-factor, variously associated with endocrine disruption, birth defects, infertility, and cancer.

Another external disease co-factor, namely electromagnetic radiation emanating from multiple sources from power lines to cell phones (as emphasized in the U.S. President's Cancer Panel Annual Report for 2008-2009) can pollute the home and work environments, and on dairy farms where 'stray voltage' affects herd health and productivity. Laboratory animal tests have demonstrated such radiation can disrupt behavior, bodily functions and the immune system.

The bioethics of Green medicine and holistic healing integrate Earth health care, human health care and animal health care. This tripartite approach to wellness and well-being is complemented by the tripartite approach to patient diagnosis and treatment of the mind-body-spirit triad. (Those who are unaware of animals' spirit or ethos have never really seen a happy, contented, playful, or spirited animal.)

Taking Responsibility

In our socio-biological evolution we have acquired a moral sensibility or conscience. When we abdicate moral responsibility for our actions, inhumanity, suffering and disease spread. People of conscience are health and environment-conscious, and conscientious consumers of foods and drugs. They have learned to question claims and assurances of governments and corporations and work to find out for themselves if there are less costly and less harmful alternatives to insure their health and well-being, and to prevent and treat disease.

But what some moral philosophers, such as Prof. Bernard Rollin with Colorado State University at Fort Collins, call Aesculapian authority is a voice not to be questioned. This principle has been embraced by organized human and animal medicine because it is believed that science is truth, which gives them a secular Papal infallibility. People must put their faith, hope and trust in science for their health and food security.

In order to be responsible consumers, parents and pet owners, we must suspend our faith and hope in some divine intercession or medical science miracle when we contemplate the threat of one or more man-made diseases of modern civilization, and become students of nutrition and health care maintenance, topics that ought to be taught from grade school and beyond.

I find the moral principle of Aesculapian authority, which means science/doctors know best, being abused by pure authoritarianism under the guise of philanthropic intentions and promises, such as those to end world hunger with pesticides and genetically engineered crops, and to cure behavioral and cognitive problems in school children with psychotropic drugs rather than addressing the many co-factors involved, notably diet and home environment. Any health authority, human or veterinary, that does not advocate a holistic, integrative approach to treatment and prevention, is to be questioned.

Although Aesculapian authority can rarely be separated from vested interests, it may be exercised with the best intentions. But the best laid plans of mice and men 'oft go awry,' like the fluoridation of municipal water which is linked to bone cancer especially in boys, and the flame-retardant chemicals in carpets to thyroid cancer in cats.

Proper disease prevention and patient treatment protocols entail consideration of endogenous and exogenous disease co-factors. Except for its focus on infectious agents, e.g. viruses and bacteria, conventional medicine's virtual dismissal of exogenous co-factors and emphasis on intervention (as with interferon, chemo-therapy, radiation, steroids and psychotropic drugs now widely dispensed to children and pets for behavioral problems) is reprehensible. Its science-base is unsound and its bioethics limited and distorted by interests vested in preserving the status quo for reasons ranging from ignorance, fear and greed; and total lack of vision and understanding. These problems and consequences stem from the multiple pathologies of anthropocentrism.

In the broader scope of things to come, the better we care for the animals and the planet, the better we will survive and prosper because we will have overcome the most pervasive co-factor of disease: Our anthropocentric, self-limited and self-limiting world view of human superiority and mastery, once wrought through magic, divination and prayer, now through medical and veterinary science and industry. We will know that the same co-factors are at work when we harm the earth because we harm ourselves, and when we abuse animals and violate their sanctity, we do no less to our own humanity and sanity. The meaning of good medicine will be recalled, and we will again speak to the plants that heal us, and to the creatures who keep us whole.

Acknowledgement. The author is grateful for the helpful suggestions of Robin Scott, MD, with earlier drafts of this chapter.

Chapter 18
Revisioning One Health

As a veterinarian I am concerned about health issues as they affect animals, causing so much suffering, as well as economic and emotional loss to people around the world. I am fully aware of the mental health benefits that a healthy, mutually symbiotic relationship with any living creature, domestic or wild, can have on a person. But I am now concerned about human health and well-being because, without any significant improvement in animals' health and well-being, be they wild tigers, whales, elephants, laboratory primates or factory farmed puppies and pigs, our own health and quality of life will continue to decline.

This basic equation

Human Well-being = Public Health+Environmental Health+Animal Health

is the holistic paradigm of integrative and complementary medicine, and is evident in the relatively new concept of the One Health or One Medicine "which seeks to improve human and animal health in the context of a shared environment." (1) It is a concept that is becoming an international academic and professional movement, no doubt stimulated by the public, environmental and animal health and welfare issues that we face today.

This One Health paradigm needs to gain greater political recognition and government support rather than continue to have to rely primarily on corporate funding of university and independent laboratory research. This reliance can create conflicts of interest, a narrowing of research and development scope, and even an erosion of objectivity and credibility, shielded from accountability and full disclosure by proprietary interests, and protected by peer review and consensus.

One Health was the theme of the 2007 American Veterinary Medical Association (AVMA). One fruit of the American Veterinary Medical Association's One Health Initiative Task Force (2) was the formation of a One Health Commission involving the collaboration of eight professional organizations including the American Medical Association (www.onehealthcommission.org). Both the World Small Animal Veterinary Association and the Federation of Veterinarians of Europe have recently embraced the One Health theme. Participants in the North

American Veterinary Education Consortium (NAVMEC) published Draft Recommendations in Oct. 2010 on core competences for all graduating veterinarians in Public health/One Health, with knowledge and expertise to help "Prevent, diagnose and control zoonotic diseases; food safety and security, emergency preparedness & response, human-animal bond benefits." I am also encouraged that the NAVMEC emphasized Multi-species clinical expertise, which included "Diagnostic, prevention and therapeutic skills, animal behavior and welfare." (Italics mine).

In April 2010, the World Organization for Animal Health, World Health Organization, Food and Agriculture Organization, United Nations Children's Fund, United Nations System Influenza Coordinator and the World Bank published a note on this tripartite concept (www.oie.int/downld/FINAL_CONCEPT_NOTE_Hanoi.pdf).

Veterinary pathologist M. J. Day (1) writes "One Health or 'One Medicine' proposes the unification of the medical and veterinary professions with the establishment of collaborative ventures in clinical care, surveillance and control of cross-species disease, education and research into disease pathogenesis, diagnosis, therapy and vaccination." In my opinion, the term 'One Medicine' is wrong because different species and individuals require different medicine when ill, but all share the One Health state of well-being when they are not ill. Also, I am concerned about Day's underscoring the importance of vaccinations, a controversial issue that is beyond the scope and intent of this section, but for details see critical reviews (2, 3, 4).

The relevance of comparative pathology and epidemiology was recognized in the 18th century by Claude Bourgelat, founder of the first veterinary school in Lyon, France in 1761, and it was British veterinarian and physician Sir John McFadyen who established the Journal of Comparative Pathology in 1888. The Section of Comparative Medicine was formed in 1923 in the Royal Society of Medicine, London. But not until 1978, with the publication of C. W. Schwabe's Wesley W. Spink Lectures on Comparative Medicine by the University of Minnesota under the book title Cattle, Priests and Comparative Medicine, was a broader scope given to the One Health concept (5).

Professor Schwabe, widely known as the father of veterinary epidemiology, brought a wealth of cross-cultural, religious, psycho-historical, and anthropological, as well as economic and environmental considerations, to the table. To quote from his University of California at Davis 2006 Obituary, "Calvin saw the world as ultimately more than the storied "one medicine"—he saw it as an ecosystem of planetary proportions constituted of interdependent civilizations and cultures, in which human history and human progress were inexorably linked with the co-evolution of the animal kingdom."

He honored my work by naming me to give the second Spink lecture series, 'Concepts in Ethology: Animal and Human Behavior,' which added further scope, and the concerns of animals' behavioral needs and related optimal care and welfare, to the nascent One Health movement (6). I was also glad to be a Founder member of the Society for Veterinary Ethology in 1966, which morphed into the International Society for Applied Animal Ethology. Now the science of animal behavior/applied ethology has become part of the curriculum in most veterinary schools. Progress indeed, as is the AVMA's decisions to recognize this field as a graduate veterinary specialty, and in 2011 to add reference to animals' welfare in their Veterinarian's Oath, coming almost thirty years after concerns over the omission of this duty in the Oath was voiced in the veterinary literature (7).

Ecosystem health, a vital component of the One Health movement, was championed by Ontario Veterinary College Dean Ole Nielsen (8), and in a later co-authored paper (9) highlighting the harmful consequences of environmental degradation, he writes: "If veterinary medicine is to remain a strong profession it must make itself more relevant to these problems. Ecosystem health management is perhaps one of the most effective vehicles for guiding veterinary medicine to address these societal imperatives." (Italics mine). This eco-veterinary perspective must be linked with ethnological considerations as essential to the practical application of veterinary bioethics in addressing wildlife conservation, environmental degradation and loss of biodiversity (10).

For there to be any significant progress in One Health/One Medicine, several barriers, political, cultural, economic, and technical, will need to be overcome. These include the major co-factors of emerging, primarily anthropogenic diseases of civilization, notably: Climate change; human population growth, mobility and morbidity, especially malnutrition; livestock numbers and densities and diseases; loss of biodiversity and invaluable biotic resources, ecosystem 'manager' and 'indicator' microorganism, plant and animal species; declining soil and fresh water quality and quantity; over-use of vaccines, antibiotics and other drugs in human patients, companion and farmed animals; pesticides and other agricultural chemicals in the mono-crop commodity farming practices of industrial agriculture, now adopting genetic engineering biotechnology and food irradiation as improved production and management practices;

industrial pollution (especially dioxins and other endocrine disruptors, carcinogens, mutagens and teratogens); and, most recently the increasing concern of electromagnetic radiation as stressed by the U.S. President's Cancer Panel 2008-2009 Annual Report. (For details go to www. environmentalhealthnews.org/ehs/news/presidents-cancer-panel).

Wildlife medicine, species conservation and management intersect with livestock health and public health concerns where wild species carry diseases transmissible to livestock (and vice versa) and humans. The 'politics of extinction' and associated wildlife habitat degradation, fragmentation and encroachment by farming, deforestation and other human activities call for more than vaccinating or exterminating infected wildlife, and funding captive breeding and reproductive research programs for endangered species. Conservation, preservation and restoration of wildlife habitat should be integral aspects of effective One Health initiatives, especially considering that most of the new 'emerging' diseases in humans originate from wild species.

However, the cultural and political resistance to limiting human and farmed animal population growth and consequential environmental degradation in developing countries limits us to a symptomatic rather than systemic approach to wildlife disease prevention and conservation. This mirrors the fragmented approach to consumer health in developed countries where a systemic One Health approach would be a threat to various industries, the livestock industry in particular with its concentrated farm animal feeding operations (CAFOs) and government funded, indiscriminate predator control programs being a prime example. Another example is the application of agrichemicals and planting of genetically engineered crops by industrial agriculture, now expanding globally in total disregard to the Precautionary Principle and to documented harm to wildlife and adverse health consequences to animals tested under controlled laboratory conditions (11).

Before One Health consortiums, commissions and courses become committed to addressing the urgent environmental and related economic crises, which affect the health and well-being of all living beings, plants and animals alike, priority funding needs to be allocated. One Health initiatives to heal and feed the world should not be adopted as primary vehicles to promote the marketing of drugs, vaccines, pesticides, agrichemicals, genetically engineered crops and livestock feed, or genetically homozygous and transgenic farmed animals, along with costly, nonsustainable, capital-intensive human and animal health care systems and standards. Those projects that incorporate a well integrated and coherent bioethical rationale should receive priority funding. This bioethical rationale goes beyond short-term, simplistic risk-benefit analyses and projections. The 'externalities' or hidden costs and 'side-effects,' direct and indirect harms, and socio-economic and ecological consequences, must be included in a total medical ecological accounting. These considerations are essential elements of the Precautionary Principle, which is based on respect for all life and needs to be applied in all of our actions.

Bioethical Considerations

Albert Schweitzer, MD, was one of the first Western physicians to advocate reverence for all life as the only antidote against the declining condition of humanity, spiritually as well as physically. He wrote "A man is ethical only when life, as such, is sacred to him, that of plants and animals as that of his fellow men, and when he devotes himself helpfully to all life that is in need of help." (12)

According to my dear friend the late Contessa Maya de Montaudouin: "The appeal for reverence and respect for life under man's stewardship is a crock of the worst kind, an empty cliché, endlessly and hypocritically repeated: nice-sounding and soothing and immediately pushed aside. Only if man can achieve a deeply felt sense of equality with all other life, will there be salvation of the planet. It is a fact that to the health of the whole we are no more valuable than the tree, the earthworm, and the blade of grass. Only if this becomes one absolute, irreversible conviction, rooted in the very depth of our soul, only then will there be salvation for all life."(13).

Respect for life (and any claim to democracy) must be absolute, unconditional, and all-encompassing–the essence of equalitarianism–or it is not respect at all. On the cusp of a global ecological, economic and health apocalypse, with spreading violence and shortages of basic, life-sustaining resources, the human species, like other endangered species on planet Earth, is being challenged to adopt new survival strategies or to face extinction. Maladaptive survival strategies include putting profits before bioethics and self before others. This new strategy calls for sound science framed in the One Health perspective that does not equate animal and human vaccinations with preventive medicine, and genetically engineered crops with sustainable agriculture and food quality and security. What is to survive of Nature, and of our better natures, is our final choice.

Being conscious that we are part of the one life, part of the same breath or spirit of Creation in a tree, a frog, or a blade of grass, we come down from the illusory hierarchical ladder of human superiority and separateness. Coming down to ground, to biological reality, we experience a sense of kinship with other living beings. This affirms our intuitive sense of the essential unity and interdependence of all life, which in turn calls upon us to give all our Earthly relations equal and fair consideration.

Such equalitarianism is the guiding principle of a new planetary politics based on an egalitarian intercultural and interspecies democracy, where we extend the Golden Rule to all beings. To have equal respect and concern for Nature and all living beings, and to live by the all-embracing Golden Rule, is ultimately enlightened self-interest.

These last three paragraphs seek to capture the global bioethics perspective of a medical doctor, oncology Professor Van Rensselaer Potter (14), who first coined the term 'bioethics.' Without the incorporation of global bioethics, more specifically articulated in veterinary bioethics (15), progress in improving the human condition will be illusory at best, even for those living under conditions of relative affluence and food security. Misguided human altruism will cause more harm than good (16).

Global bioethics calls us to give equally fair consideration to three spheres of moral concern: Human well-being (rights and interests); nonhuman (animal and plant) well-being (rights and interests); and, environmental well-being (co-evolved biodiversity and ecosystemic integrity and sustainability). Global bioethics calls us to be accountable for our actions and appetites in relation to these three spheres, and to examine how well our society, politics, professions, laws, economies (industry and commerce), and religious, educational and other secular traditions and institutions, are in accord with the bioethical principles that unify these three spheres in the light and language of compassion, humility, and respect for the sanctity of life.

As food, fuel and water scarcity and costliness spread and intensify globally, along with rising populations and the scourges of corrupted governments and failing economies and employment markets, the kind of agriculture and medicine and all the associated inputs of seeds, vaccines, pesticides, antibiotics, and costly equipment for harvesting and processing, diagnosing and treating, need to be examined from the One Health, One World perspective of global bioethics. It must be noted that the Western diet has triggered an obesity epidemic and escalating public costs and suffering from associated diseases. I reason, from this perspective, the necessity of the abolition of CAFOs and the adoption of ecological and organically certified farming practices, including sustainable biofuel production (not from GM corn), along with integrative holistic veterinary and human medicine.

The triad of human, animal and environmental health calls for the application of global bioethics in determining how best to repair and manage the co-dependencies and mutually enhancing symbioses at all levels of the biotic community. Hence, the involvement of holistic healing and integrative medicine in the political, legal and economic triad of government, corporate and public responsibility and accountability is inevitable. This is especially true when it comes to how nonhuman life and the natural environment are regarded and treated.

The abolition of what many term vivisection—performing experiments on animals to test new cosmetics and other consumables, chemical compounds and drugs to primarily treat diseases of our own making which are preventable, and even testing military weapons—is long overdue. But studying animal diseases, their treatment and prevention, including those transmissible to humans, is sound science and good medicine, being ethically justifiable when there is a mutuality of benefit for humans and animals alike under the banners of integrative medicine and One Health.

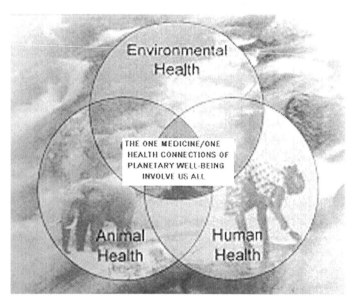

Figure 18-1. The One Health Connections for Planetary Well-being

Summary

In summary, the holistic healing and integrative medicine perspectives of the One Health address the many co-factors of disease within the triads of human, animal and environment; body, mind and spirit; patient, environment and pathogen; and, genetics, epigenetics and nutrition (of body, mind and spirit). Dis-ease triggering co-factors in the stress triad of excess, that is, deficiency and imbalance in gene expression, nutrition, and psycho-physical homeostasis reflecting quality of life, are challenges that differ qualitatively and quantitatively from species to species, individual to individual, and time and place. Integrative holistic medicine incorporates the metaphysical perception of the universal in the particular and the particular in the universal as an antidote to reductionist scientific paradigms and economic determinism being applied in deciding best treatment protocols. Vaccinating and medicating malnourished children and animals housed under stressful conditions, without simultaneously addressing local food-sufficiency needs, better housing and lower densities and numbers, is a popular treatment protocol today—but it has to warrant closer scrutiny in particular.

Many crop and farm animal diseases are caused or aggravated by farming practices that cause 'agricologenic' diseases in crops and 'domestogenic' production-related diseases in farmed animals. Some of these diseases are being recognized under the new paradigm of One Health (such as moldy grain aflatoxins and foodborne illnesses connected with some 3,000 deaths and 128,000 hospitalizations annually in the US). Their prevention means alternative farming practices, which are basically organic and humane, but alternatives are a threat to those vested interests that profit from selling products to combat agricologenic and domestogenic diseases of plants and animals in industrial systems of production. An AVMA survey of veterinary school graduates in 2009 found that only two percent of the graduating class planned to work in the food animal sector, where some 28.7 million pounds of antibiotics were sold for use in food producing animals in the US in 2009, according to the Animal Health Institute (17). Clearly the problems of farmed animal health and welfare and food safety and security will be compounded by a lack of veterinarians in this sector. Furthermore, this sector of the food industry is a major contributor to climate change, loss of biodiversity, environmental degradation, wildlife diseases, and a host of zoonotic diseases and diet-related health problems in humans. We must provide incentives and reasons to encourage graduates to go where they are needed, to address the problems of industrial animal production or to change the paradigm.

The sciences and technologies of conventional veterinary and human medicine and industrial agriculture may be morally laudable, but they are inadequate to help improve the human condition, especially when driven by the mammonite imperatives of profitability and corporate hegemony, notably by the pharmaceutical industry (18). The increasing recognition and acceptance of the principles and praxis of One Health by the world's leading human and animal health organizations, coupled with a failing health care system in most countries, and with rising public demand for improved food, water and air quality, along with planetary CPR— conservation, preservation and restoration—give some grounds for hope. But, that will be a premature sentiment if the outcome does not herald a post-anthropocentric age based on the global bioethical imperatives of giving all sentient beings equal and fair consideration, and respect for the natural environment that sustains us all.

The consequences of human engineering of mind and matter, beliefs and values, chemicals and genes, entire ecosystems and human and non-human communities, have helped give us this world we have inherited, but which we should not be passing on if we care for the well-being of future generations. When such trans-species and intergenerational concerns of global bioethics become part of a global One Health movement, we may then secure a more viable future for the Earth community.

ADDENDA

A-1. Ethology & Bioethics

Remember that Konrad Lorenz once said, "Before you can really study an animal, you must first love it." We have to recognize that necessary connection. In a shamanic sense, through empathy we can connect with and be one with the animal, like Martin Buber's "I-Thou" experience that he described with a beloved horse. The taboo of anthropomorphizing animals is thus transcended, possibly through a kind of counter-transference where, given sufficient intimacy with the animal, we zoomorphize ourselves: we "morph" into the animal's consciousness, being able to anticipate her actions, understand her intentions, needs, and motivational state.

In some respects ethology is like meditation, focusing on one or more animals until the door of perception begins to open. The first intimation of this is being able to anticipate/predict their actions and reactions, and in a sense, therefore, read the animals' minds and become them. Since most animals are readily able to do this with each other it should not be so difficult for us. Our major obstacles are anthropocentric conditioning, and the ignorance arising from those cultural values and attitudes toward other animals who are regarded as our inferiors in both sentience and sapience.

Ethology is close in its scientific methodology to phenomenology and existential psychology. Behavioral socio-ecology looks at adaptive processes, their ontogeny and phylogeny, as does cognitive ethology that explores the animals' umwelt or perceptual world, while sociobiology is traditionally more genetically deterministic.

The existential, phenomenological approach of ethology, which some critics do not regard as scientific, is one of observation and description. As one of the other founding fathers of ethology, Nobel Laureate Nikko Tinbergen once said, "When you put two animals together, you have an experiment." Observation and identification of behaviors and detailed description in various contexts lead to the construction of an "ethogram"—a listing of the animal's repertoire of behavioral action patterns, displays and vocalizations in various contexts and emotional/ motivational states, like sexual (including courtship), parental, agonistic, allelomimetic (group coordinated), self-care, mutual care, eliminative, ingestive, exploratory, investigative (including social), hunting, predator defense, den or nest-making, and play behavior – including self-play, play with another (social play), and play with an inanimate object that in some species can link with tool-using behavior.

Some behaviors are highly ritualistic in that they are predictable, stereotypic fixed-action patterns. These are called displays and their ritualistic form helps reduce ambiguity and therefore misunderstanding. When a dog growls and snaps, you know his intentions and [maybe] the cause of such an agonistic display. But since similar ritualistic signals or fixed-action patterns can be displayed in different contexts — a dog will snarl and snap when the context is playful rather than threatening – we learn through the ethogram that animals are aware of context: in one context the threat is serious, in another it is not. This gives us insight into animal consciousness and awareness and of their ability to "ethologize" or interpret each other's behavior, motivational state, needs, wants and intentions. We find elements of humor, deception, misunderstanding, mirroring or mimicry, and altruism in how they communicate and relate.

The objectifying (and objectional) Cartesian/Newtonian umwelt mechanomorphizes the animal, reducing complex and context-related behavior and consciousness to numerical, statistically verifiable probabilities. Subjected to Darwinian/sociobiological selective filtering, the adaptive, evolutionary and genetic determinants of what and how animals do what they do, and when, may be deduced or induced. Yet such deductive and inductive reasoning that imposes on the animal anthropocentric projections, like intentionality and purposiveness in terms of survival and adaptability and genetic investment in mate or offspring, may lead to erroneous conclusions. For example, many studies of animal play conclude that play helps refine hunting and fighting skills or escape from predators, the sheer joy and bonding function of play, including interspecies play, being off the conceptual screen.

Ethology enables us to better understand the ethos or spirit of animals. With better understanding of their behavior, we can improve methods and standards of husbandry or animal care. We can also gain insight, especially through studies of their care-giving and care-soliciting (epimeletic and et-epimeletic) behaviors, of their capacity for empathy, altruism and elemental moral and ethical sensibility. It's all very well to put a Darwinian/sociobiological spin on such behavior, but in my mind it should move us to consider the moral status we give to nonhuman animals and to the ethical, philosophical and socio-economic ramifications of animal rights.

Empathy in animals and altruistic behavior give us biological evidence of an evolutionary process of increasing social and mental complexity converging and giving rise to an innate moral sensibility and capacity to make ethical decisions for the good of the pack (in the wolf) and of the Earth community (for the human), where self-interest through empathy becomes synonymous with the interests of others. Altruistic behavior is thus the most enlightened form of selfishness.

There is one human quality that animal studies may never be able to shed comparative, biological and evolutionary light on, and that is our imagination, animal play notwithstanding. The power of imagination to manifest materially or behaviorally—ideas ("mnemes," acting culturally like genes) that we mentally conceive—is a power, like our power of dominion, that demands more of us than the "biophilia" and "conciliation" of Harvard Biologist E. O. Wilson.

As for the neo-Darwinian view of the human species being the supreme, most highly evolved being on Earth, according to a family friend, Darwin used to write on his hand a daily reminder "not superior." The essence of his evolutionary theory is more subtle than the fundamentalist vernacular Darwinism of human superiority and of competition and survival of the fittest. He drew attention to cooperation and interspecies co-evolution, that contradicts the social Darwinism of the industrial age that puts humans at the top of an Aristotelian great chain of being; and that interprets evolution as increasing technological perfection, industrial growth, and scientific progress, even reasoning that genetic engineering is a natural evolutionary progression for the human species, and that being natural is therefore neither immoral nor unethical.

Darwin's view of cooperation resonates with Peter Kropotkin's thesis of mutual aid. He coined the term anarchy to describe the absence of a ruling species and of a hierarchy in the ecosystem of Russian steppes. The term holarchy may now be more appropriate considering the negative connotations of anarchism.

The ethos, spirit or nature of animals, is intimately linked ontogenetically and phylogenetically with their telos, or purpose in being; and with their ecos, the ecosystem environment in which they have co-evolved with other species in a mutually enhancing, sustainable and regenerative "holarchy" of interdependence.

The intimate linkages between ethos, telos, and ecos have been disrupted by the domestication effects on animals' ethos and telos. The same may be said for the post-gatherer-hunter civilization effects on the human ethos and telos, of agrarianism, sedentarism, urbanization and industrialization. The profound ecological, environmental, social and psychological consequences on human species are part of the "price of progress," as some see it, or of human adaptation and evolution. But all to what end?

The etymology of human implies our origin from humus, invoking humility and humaneness. If we are to learn anything from animals wild and domestic, it is that we are animals too, affected for better or for worse by what we have done to the Earth and all who dwell therein. Through the animals we can discern the better attributes of their ethos that make us human – empathy, compassion, altruism, playfulness, curiosity, adaptability and creativity, attributes that are so often lacking in society today.

The Jesuit priest and paleontologist Teilhard de Chardin saw evolution as a creative convergence of two axes – consciousness and complexity – that more recently has been cast in a creative, cosmogenic process by Thomas Berry, who urges us to see the universe as a communion of subjects and not as a collection of objects.

It calls for the recovery of our animal heritage of empathy and altruism; a redefinition or clarification of what it means to be human, and the incorporation of bioethics into our daily lives to help restore the linkages – or sacred connections – between ethos, telos, and the Earth Mother of us all.

A-2. The Euthanasia Question

When a fellow being is suffering without hope of relief and recovery, those who care will opt for mercy killing (euthanasia). Euthanasia is unacceptable in some cultures and religious traditions because to deliberately kill another being, such as a "holy cow," is taboo. This has less to do with the life and plight of the animal than with the shame of making oneself "impure" by killing another. Self-interest, in this instance, takes precedence over compassionate action. Such inaction (letting the animal continue to suffer) is more than cowardice. It is the essence of hypocrisy when euthanasia is equated not with compassion but with violence, disobedience to some religious doctrine (like ahimsa — nonharming), and personal defilement. Any cultural or religious moral principle like ahimsa, other than compassion itself, cannot be absolute, since there are extenuating circumstances, i.e., situational ethics. But just as not killing an animal out of compassion can be a purely selfish choice, I have been in situations where my decision to euthanize an animal was difficult to separate from my own empathic suffering. Putting the animal out of its misery would put an end to my own burden of suffering for the animal. It is difficult therefore to be compassionate and at the same time sufficiently detached to be able to make the right decision free of self-interest.

I recall one instance in India, treating a Pomeranian dog "Snowflake" who had lost most of the skin on her back—about one third of her surface area—from an accidental scalding. My first reaction, while cleaning the massive wound, was to consider euthanizing her. But strangely, she seemed to be in less pain than I, and with her indefatigable spirit and will to live, combined with intensive wound care and love, she healed completely in 3 months.

We should adopt neither a sanguine nor an abolitionist attitude toward euthanasia. The compassionate middle-ground between these extremes can be difficult to establish, as for instance in India where appeals to reason and compassion with regard to animal euthanasia can evoke violent opposition. It is indeed tragic when abandoned cows starve to death and when homeless dogs are neutered and released only to suffer a hopeless existence on busy city streets before they are killed by traffic or are rounded up by municipal dog-catchers to be killed by electrocution or with injections of strychnine and cyanide. The western humanitarians' policy of humanely euthanizing all homeless dogs especially in cities (as distinct from those dogs who have homes or belong to the village community and roam free) is anathema to many of their counterparts in the East.

Surrounded by suffering, we can become desensitized to it. The attitude of live and let live can then have cruel consequences when responsible euthanasia is taboo.

A-3. Unwarranted Surgical Alterations of Companion Animals

Feline Phalangectomy

Many veterinarians in the U.S. routinely de-claw young cats. It's part of the package when they come in to be spayed/neutered. Many cats suffer as a consequence. The operation entails more than simply removing the claws, (onychectomy) under general anesthesia. It entails removal of the first digit (phalangectomy). It's like you having your toes and fingers removed at the first joint, i.e. a radical phalangectomy.

Cats are very dexterous, and this operation essentially eliminates their dexterity, greatly reducing their behavioral repertoire when it comes to grasping and holding. It also hampers their ability to groom and scratch themselves normally. Their ability and self-confidence when it comes to climbing and general agility are similarly crippled. Their first line of defense—their retractable claws— is eliminated, which could make some cats more anxious and defensive.

De-clawed cats tend to walk abnormally back on their heels rather than on their entire pads because of the chronic pain at the end of their severed fingers and toes. They often develop chronic arthritis and as the front toe pads shrink, chronic bone infections are common.

Many cats find it painful to use the litter box, develop a conditioned aversion to using the box, and become unhousebroken. This is why many de-clawed cats are put up for adoption or are euthanized. They may also bite more, and become defensive when handled because their paws are hurting and infected.

I strongly advise all prospective cat owners, and those people with cats who are contemplating having the entire first digit—not simply the claw—removed surgically from their cats' paws—never to have this operation performed on their felines.

Cats need their claws to be cats, and the routine surgical amputation of all their first digits is considered unthinkable in the UK and many other countries where people love and respect their cats. They know that properly handled and socialized cats quickly learn not to scratch people, and will learn to enjoy using a scratch post and not destroy upholstered furniture.

According to the Paw Project (www.pawproject.org), de-clawing has become extremely common in the US and Canada in the past three decades. Before that time, it was rarely performed. In most countries, de-clawing is considered unethical and is not performed by veterinarians. De-clawing is illegal in many countries, including Austria, Croatia, Malta, Israel, Belgium, Bulgaria, Cyprus, Czech Republic, Denmark, Finland, France, Germany, Greece, Lithuania, Luxembourg, Norway, Portugal, Romania, Sweden, Switzerland, and Turkey.

I wrote the following letter on this topic to my colleagues was published in the Journal of the American Veterinary Medical Association, Feb. 15, 2006, pages 503-504.

Dear Sir,

The article by Drs. Curicio, Bidwell, Bohart, and Hauptman (JAVMA, January 1, 2006, pp. 65-680) provides an "Evaluation of signs of postoperative pain and complications after forelimb onychectomy in cats receiving buprenorphine alone or with bupivacaine administered as a four-point regional nerve block." While the consideration given to pain alleviation in this surgical procedure is necessary and laudable, the ethics of performing this procedure as a routine practice to the extent that almost a quarter of the cat population in the US, (14 million) is declawed, according to these authors, surely need to be examined. This is especially pertinent considering the evidence of the painful nature of this procedure, and associated postoperative complications of chronic pain, infection, and suffering. Surely the justifications for performing forelimb onychectomies trivialize concern for cats' welfare and psychological well being. Part of being a cat is to have claws. Out of respect for the nature of cats and their basic behavioral requirements in the confined domestic environment, caring and responsible cat owners effectively train their cats to use scratch-posts, scratch-boards and carpeted "condos" rather than resort to routine declawing, that amounts to a mutilation for convenience.

As a profession, are we not giving a mixed message to the public in advocating companion animal health and welfare on the one hand, and not abandoning such practices that are considered unethical by veterinarians and their clients in many other countries?
Michael W. Fox, D.Sc., Ph.D., B.Vet.Med, M.R.C.V.S.

Further Observations
From the perspectives of naturalistic philosophy and ethics the cat's ritualistic claw-scratching to mark the territorial domain is a vital practice that helps cats relax and discharge pent up energies. Ethologically, cats' need to scratch suitable vertical and semi-vertical objects with their claw-marks and paw-pad pheromones is motivated by the desire for safety and security in a regularly marked, familiar territory. Scratch-post sites are tied to self-identity and recognition: self-awareness.

I have observed feral and free-roaming cats and indoor cats all engaging in scratch-post-marking behavior, and to take this ritual away from them by de-clawing is to rob them both physically and psychologically of their first line of defense in a potentially hostile world; and of their ability to even be able to mark their territories effectively. So many begin to urine-spray-mark, or show behavioral changes associated with increased fear and vulnerability. Unable to even move without discomfort, forever unable to hold various objects securely, yet with exquisite tenderness with their claws, many de-clawed felines become depressed, lethargic, and just want to eat and sleep which is good for neither man nor beast.

Cats are fastidious self-groomers, and they need their claws to be able to groom themselves properly. Unable to groom themselves, cats become more irritable, tense, depressed.

These problems are compounded by the chronic pain that many de-clawed cats suffer, and show lameness and abnormal vertebral and postural misalignments due to paw-pad pain from abnormal weight distribution on certain pads, and also from chronic inflammation, post-surgical infection, chronic arthritis and osteomyelitis, and contractions of the flexor tendons.

Such physical and psychological crippling of cats has become an accepted cultural norm. But such perverse defilement of the cat's nature, her ethos, such mutilation, rationalized disfigurement as a necessary convenience, is a sad reflection of our humanity, or lack thereof. Both must be addressed, and all veterinary colleges censored where de-clawing is taught to students with the expectation that this would be a routine source of income because of public demand, and if vets were not around to do it properly, many people would resort to using wire-cutters.

Conclusions

Performing phalangectomies on cats as a routine preventive measure, just in case they might scratch people or damage furniture, is a service of convenience to cat owners that I consider professionally unethical for veterinarians to offer and perform as a routine procedure on all cats that come through their doors. It is nothing less than a mutilation that takes away from cats an integral part of what makes them cats—a form of physical deprivation with often profound behavioral and psychological ramifications, the risks of which far outweigh the benefits to uninformed cat owners and lovers. Many veterinarians argue that it is a life-saving procedure because otherwise cats that might damage furniture or scratch their owners are often euthanized if they are not de-clawed. I see this as engaging in self-serving emotional blackmail, financial interests notwithstanding.

Dr. Ron Gaskin, who runs a veterinary practice in Shakopee, Minnesota, and operates on de-clawed cats to help correct crippling post-declawing flexor tendon contractions, in a recent e-mail to me wrote:

"The shifting of weight from front paws to back paws can lead to lower back muscle spasms. These back cramps hurt.

Idea: We need a gait analysis recording of these declawed cats! We put it in objective computerized form everyone will believe!

Cat owners looking for a fast convenient fix to cat scratching are also quick to get rid of a cat that bites or does not use the litter box. The declawing and surrender of a cat are deeply related."

Canine Ear-Cropping & Tail-Docking

I advise people who are planning to get a purebred puppy like a Schnauzer, Boxer, or Doberman Pincher, for dog's sake to tell the breeder not to cut off the tail of the pup they want. And when they get the puppy with a tail, don't have the next cruel and unnecessary mutilation done on the poor creature, namely, ear-cropping.

I advise against having either of these procedures done on any pup, not just because they are outlawed in the UK as unwarranted and unethical cosmetic alterations. They also cause harm, and can have long-tem health and behavioral problems.

First, consider why dogs have tails. Regardless of the fact that some mutants have no tails at birth, dogs need and use their tails as one means of communication, especially for making their intentions clear to other dogs. Tails are used to signal friendliness, submission, fear, playfulness, dominance, and threats. They are even used as play-toys by pups pulling and leaping on their mothers' tails, who will twitch them to stimulate their offspring. Thick and furry tails can provide warmth and comfort to tuck into on a chilly night, and a strong tail can help provide counterbalance when running and turning fast. So why cut them off because it is some 'breed standard'? Change the standards.

Dogs with docked tails sometimes become almost psychotic because there is a painful abscess on the tip of their tails where the skin did not heal properly over the amputated tail vertebra. Bone infection may set in, necessitating further amputation of the tail.

Other unfortunate dogs do seem to become really psychotic when they compulsively chase their tails and have bouts of chewing them bloody. There's no infection involved. The cause of the extreme suffering may be due to a phantom-limb effect, or to what is called an amputation neuroma. This is an inflamed and swollen severed nerve-ending that pulses pain-impulses into the heart and soul of the poor dog.

Second, consider why dogs have ears. A normal dog's ear, with complex muscles that enable dogs to move their ears independently and into different positions, not only plays a role in enhancing dogs' hearing ability and ability to locate the direction of sounds, but is also an integral part of dogs' communication repertoire. Like the tail, different ear positions mean different things when combined with various facial expressions, body postures, and vocal sounds. Dogs with erect, cropped ears are hampered in this regard, and may be seen as more threatening by other dogs—and people too. How does this affect a naturally gentle dog, to be perceived as aggressive or dangerous? While assessing animal concerns with Masai cattle people in East Africa, after seeing that some of their dogs had cropped ears, I asked them why they had done so. They told me it was done to make chosen dogs 'more fierce'.

Psychological problems can arise following ear cropping, especially in dogs that developed infections along the sliced, sutured edges of their ears. Often such dogs have to go in for more surgery, and have their hot, suppurating, and painful ears cleaned, dressed and bandaged for days. Frequently when one or both ears do not stand up as hoped for, the poor pup has to go in for additional plastic surgery or wear uncomfortable ear-splints for weeks.

The net result is suffering, and fear that result in some dogs becoming head-shy, either cringing, or even snapping when anyone comes close and reaches to pat or stroke them on their heads. So rather than becoming 'more fierce,' some dogs will become more fearful or unreliable, especially around strangers. Of course many pups have no problems with their ears, but you can never be sure if they won't. So why run the risk, and unanticipated costs?

Clearly injurious, far from harmless, and not without serious consequences, the practices of dog tail-docking and ear cropping should be regarded as unnecessary mutilations that should be seen as cruelties under animal protection laws, statutes, and welfare standards. Breed clubs should set a date after which, any dog born after that date, cannot enter a dog show without a full tail and uncropped ears. And all veterinarians should give up their income from ear cropping to the higher calling of our profession: And that is to prevent animal disease and suffering wherever and whenever we can.

I have seen more than one Schnauzer, Boxer and Doberman with their entire tails and uncropped ears. They looked different, of course, from a distance, but behaviorally and in spirit they were still true to their breeds. I think they looked magnificent; and they were as happy as their human companions were proud! (For details see M.W. Fox, 2010, A Veterinarian's Personal Manifesto at www.twobitdog.com/DrFox/).

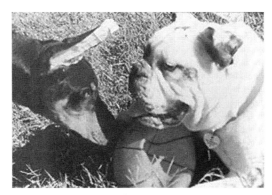

Figure A-3-1. Doberman with recent ear crop. Bulldog bred for extreme traits (pushed-in face, large head). Both practices should be abolished.

A-4. Concerning Puppy & Kitten Breeding Mills

Since my first investigations of commercial dog breeding facilities and practices in the Midwest in the early 1970's, commerce in purebred and 'designer' (cross-breed) dogs, and purebred cats has expanded in many farming states. Brood-bitches, stud dogs and litters of puppies are generally treated like commodities; no different from other livestock, such as pigs, chickens, and fur-ranch foxes and mink. Over three decades ago inhumane breeding practices and conditions were widespread, and they have not been improved upon over the intervening years in spite of government (USDA/APHIS) inspections and licensing schemes and purported AKC (American Kennel Club) inspections. Some state authorities still see nothing wrong with applying the same minimal health and welfare standards for how producers raise and treat their livestock and poultry, to puppy and kitten mill commercial breeding facilities.

On large commercial breeding facilities there is inadequate human contact and socialization of mass-produced puppies and kittens, leading potentially to emotionally unstable, unreliable, even unsafe animals. Their parent 'breeding stock' can suffer their entire lives from lack of consistent and caring human contact. This is compounded by living in a literal prison cage or wire run, often in extremely noisy and crowded conditions where sanitation, clean water, and adequate food and shelter may all be deficient to some degree.

All this means animal stress and distress, which impairs their immune systems leading to increased susceptibility to diseases. Some of these are zoonotic diseases transmissible to humans. They include round worms (Toxacara) that can cause blindness in children, to ringworm that can ravage a family and Toxoplasmosis that can cause human

fetal abnormalities and birth defects. Other diseases that can take hold
in unsanitary facilities and stressed animals and be transmitted from
infected puppies and kittens to humans (children, the elderly, and others
with impaired immune systems being especially vulnerable), include:
Salmonellosis, Campylobacter enteritis, Leptospirosis, Blastomycosis,
Histoplasmosis, Giardiasis, Echinococcosis, and Sarcoptic mange.

Pups and kittens whose mothers were chronically stressed during
pregnancy, and environmental influences, especially diet, and quality of
human contact or lack thereof, during their first few weeks of life can
suffer alterations in the 'wiring' of their nervous, endocrine and other
body systems. This is called epigenetics, a recent branch of human and
veterinary medicine and that was an integral aspect of my first doctoral
dissertation (published in 1971 by the University of Chicago Press, entitled
'Integrative Development of Brain and Behavior in the Dog.'). This in
part accounts for the high veterinary bills people find themselves paying
because of the chronic health problems afflicting their puppy and kitten-
mill produced animal companions

Another reason for the plethora of health problems in pure-
bred animals is because of the low 'hybrid vigor' and higher incidence
of genetic and developmental abnormalities, hereditary diseases, and
behavioral problems ranging from extreme shyness to unpredictable
aggression and hyperactivity syndrome. Large scale commercial breeders—
anyone with say more than six breeding animals—cannot follow up
through the marketing matrix to determine the quality of their produce.
They have no system of progeny testing, which means keeping records of
all the health and behavioral problems of the puppies and kittens that they
are marketing that could be traced to a 'defective' bitch or stud dog. It is
inexcusable that the AKC, that opposes any legislation like this Bill, should
actually profit from selling pedigree registration papers to the unwitting
purchasers of puppy mill puppies.

Additional stress is placed on the offspring when they are shipped
out, shortly after the stress of being weaned that is coupled additional
stress on their immune systems by being wormed and given a cocktail of
vaccinations. Such treatments can lead to life-long sickness and suffering.
Kittens and puppies should not be shipped any distance more than a two-
four-hour journey in a climate-controlled vehicle and then only after they
have passed the sensitive period of development that in the dog is around 8
weeks of age, and possibly one or two weeks later in kittens. 'Locally bred
and locally purchased' animals could be sold at an earlier age, around 6-7
weeks of age for puppies, and 7-8 weeks for kittens, provided the distances

they must travel are within the two-four hour range.

The 'breeding stock' not only suffer a life of extreme confinement on the typical puppy and kitten mill facility: They also suffer the stress of repeated pregnancies one heat cycle after another with no rest and recovery after raising a litter. Most are bred, for cost-saving, on their first heat, at an age when they are not yet even fully grown and physiologically ready to bear offspring. No conscientious breeder would ever consider adopting such a stressful practice.

All who respect the nature and beauty of cats and who appreciate how dogs have contributed to the well-being of humanity since before the beginning of recorded history, would give nothing less than unequivocal support for legislation that would help reduce the suffering and improve the health and well-being of dogs and cats used for commercial breeding purposes, and their helpless offspring. Their health is also a significant public health issues that no responsible legislator or governmental agency can ignore.

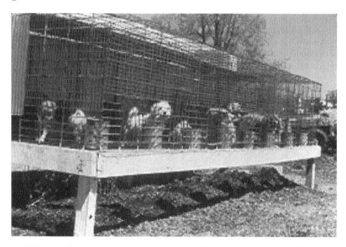

Figure A-4-1. *A typical puppy mill where some breed dogs spend their entire lives (Photo by an undercover investigator)*

A-5. Concerning the Outdoor Chaining/Tethering of Dogs

(From a statement by Dr. Fox in support of a State Bill in North Carolina to outlaw keeping dogs for most of their lives tethered outdoors—a Bill needed to be put into legislation in most States across the US).

The common practice in many communities, where it is not yet forbidden under local ordinance, or is accepted with strictly specified time-restrictions and effective inspections and enforcement by animal control authorities, of keeping one or more dogs restrained on a chain or other material such as a wire cable or rope, is unacceptable for several reasons. Regardless of whether the dog has adequate shade and shelter and is provided water and sufficient freedom of movement so as not to become tangled or hung, being kept out on a chain/tether affects the flight and critical distance reactions of dogs.

The longer and more frequently a dog is kept outdoors under such restraint, the more the dog's behavior will change. Normal flight and critical (attack) distances are disrupted by such restraint, making friendly dogs more likely to become aggressive when approached by a stranger; turning timid dogs into so-called fear-biters; and aggressive dogs into dangerous animals.

The longer and more frequently a dog is so restrained, the more behavioral abnormalities or pathologies are likely to develop from a combination of being physically, behaviorally and psychologically confined to a life-space dictated by the length of the constraining tether. Signs of behavioral pathology, that are indicative of stress and emotional distress, include stereotypic (repetitive, obsessive-compulsive) pacing, spinning, running to and fro, frenzied chewing to get free; and displacement behaviors such as digging, and excessive self-licking, even to the point of self-mutilation. Many such dogs bark and whine incessantly, resulting in cruel retribution when neighbors complain, or no less cruel surgical de-vocalization.

The suffering of dogs chained outdoors, extremes of weather notwithstanding, is compounded by the fact that the dog is a pack animal and wants to be with his or her family and 'master' in the house. Such emotional/social deprivation is in many instances intensified by the outdoor dog seeing one or more pet dogs in the house who are never chained outside.

Nobel prize laureate the late Dr. Konrad Lorenz, and author of the bestselling book *Man Meets Dog*, would insist that these tethered outside dogs, who should be inside with their human pack, manifest a pathological disruption of their ethos or behavior, meaning a total distortion of their conceptual, emotional and social space as a result of being confined to a universe defined by the length of their chains.

This can make for a dangerous dog, turning a gentle dog into one that is more likely to attack; and a trustworthy and friendly dog into a public safety risk, especially toward children.

Dogs that are routinely kept chained/tethered outdoors result in the most frequently reported public nuisance complaint for incessant and uncontrolled barking, and worse: Prolonged chaining/tethering can result in permanent changes in dogs' temperaments, making them hyper-excitable and unpredictable when set free. I have been consulted on several occasions, and served as an expert witness, for dog-bite cases involving children especially, but also adults, who were injured, in some cases fatally, by their own or neighborhood dogs. The best preventives are proper rearing, socialization, care and handling of dogs, coupled with public education and effective enforcement of anti-cruelty and animal protection laws that include the prohibition of keeping dogs outdoors permanently chained/tethered.

I would concur with Dr. Lorenz, and add that if dogs are to be outdoors they should be free to run and play, ideally with members of their own kind rather than being alone, in a safe, confined area, for short periods of time during the day.

In conclusion, from the perspectives not of tradition, custom, or cultural values, but of veterinary bioethics and animal behavior science, the prolonged tethering of dogs outdoors is inhumane, and unethical. It is likely to turn a good dog into an aggressive dog, and a healthy dog into a neurotic and emotionally unstable one. The practice, therefore, of people tying their dogs up outside for hour upon hour should be prohibited by law in the name of compassion, and in the spirit of a civil society that equates social progress with the humane treatment of all animals within the community.

Postscript

This 2007 Bill in North Carolina, like similar Bills in other States, was defeated, in large part because of the effective lobbying of the American Kennel Club, for whom the suffering of hundreds of thousands of dogs every day is of less concern than protecting the vested interests of those who find perverse profit in keeping dogs tied up outdoors most if not all of their lives.

A-6. A Response to the Bateson Independent Inquiry into Dog Breeding in the U.K. (www.dogbreedinginquiry.com)

Anyone who cares about dogs cannot ignore this document and its long overdue recommendations. As a concerned veterinarian involved for many years advocating attention be given to the main issues in the Bateson report, I am glad that this document once more puts before the consumer-public and pedigree dog community the long recognized problems and remedies that undermine the health and welfare of pedigree dogs— But it is incomplete.

Professor Bateson urges the 'veterinary profession as a whole to support enforcement authorities, help educate the public, and lead a shift towards a preventative approach to dog health'. Without even mentioning the role of manufactured pet foods, vaccinations and other veterinary treatments which have iatrogenic consequences which underlie a variety of diseases in particular breeds, and the risks of same to the larger dog population, this report is of limited value at best in helping educate the public and fostering a preventive approach to canine health and well-being.

Just looking at 'breeding practices' and treatment of show dogs and breeding stock, might amount to a cover-up, which Bateson will say is untrue since his brief 'was to consider whether the health and welfare of dogs, and particularly pedigree dogs, is affected and/or can be improved, by reference to the registration, breeding and showing of dogs" (Vet Rec. Jan 23, p 91, 2010).

This report may make those with vested interests—from those in science to those involved in the commerce of dog breeding, feeding and health care, as well as those involved in regulatory authority, feel better. But I doubt that many dogs will be better for it in the long -term. I am pessimistic because any real change, not in the commoditization of dogs but in what they are being fed, vaccinated and otherwise treated with may be fought from every quarter.

A review of inherited disorders in purebred dogs published in the British Veterinary Journal (2010, Vol 183: 39-45) will serve as a consumer alert and a clear appeal to breeders to be ever more vigilant in weeding out these problems which can mean a life of suffering and much expense. In a review of the top 50 breeds registered with the UK Kennel Club a total of 312 inherited disorders were identified, the German shepherd dog having the most—58 different disorders. Disorders affecting the largest number of breeds were hypothyroidism (43 breeds); hereditary adult onset cataracts (38 breeds), and progressive retinal atrophy (35 breeds). (For an earlier review by the American Association of Veterinarians for Animal Rights, check my website www.twobitdog.com/DrFox/)

The status quo has been preserved to a regrettable degree by this report not addressing the health and welfare of dogs from a more holistic science and evidence- based medical perspective which would not exclude such critical factors as nutritional genomics and epigenetics, vaccinosis— adverse reactions to vaccinations—and the genetics of iatrogenic, treatment-induced illnesses. In sum, the welfare of pedigree dogs entails more than what the Bateson report addresses. None of his veterinary advisors seems to have raised this issue, since Prof. Bateson's report barely mentions the fact that adverse reactions to vaccines and certain food ingredients especially common in certain purebreds are also prevalent in the larger canine population as well.

But in all fairness, the information which might have lead to this Inquiry unearthing the health problems in pedigree, pure-bred and other dogs that are associated with manufactured foods and vaccinosis was actually denied by the British pet insurance sector. In one key instance cited in the report the insurance company 'refused point blank to share any data under any circumstances on grounds of commercial confidentiality."

Consider the anthropogenic chemical risks in the environment of any dog, first exposed *in utero* as an embryo, and then as a puppy exposed after birth via the mother's milk to what she was given to eat could mean a lifetime of allergies or early death from cancer. That dog may be susceptible to chemical damage of certain genes responsible for the normal functioning of the nervous, endocrine, immune, digestive or other body system or process. Nutrition influences gene expression, and cannot be ignored when looking at the health problems of dogs from an integrative approach that considers etiological demographics, environmental factors pre-and postnatal, and not just hereditary factors. That the Bateson Inquiry was denied access to such relevant date by the UK pet health insurance industry is shameful indeed.

To blame the genes and alter or eugenically eliminate them, or develop drugs to silence or activate them, is more profitable than correcting external, anthropogenic causes. Such bio-molecular endeavors are touted as progress, and genetic determinism becomes the new myth of scientific reductionism and the hope to feed and heal the world.

An independent inquiry into the resolution and prevention of diseases simply through feeding biologically-appropriate whole-food diets to sick dogs and cats being fed the kinds of processed foods the major multinationals like Procter & Gamble, Colgate-Palmolive, Mars

(MasterFoods), and Nestle Inc. are marketing, and which veterinarians are selling world-wide, is surely needed. Then pet owners may benefit doubly by not eating the kinds of products also being manufactured for them to eat and drink.

A-7. Cloning Dogs & Cats

Goats, sheep, cows, pigs, rabbits, mules, horses, deer, cats and mice have been cloned for commercial and biomedical purposes. In August, 2005, the first dog was cloned, an Afghan hound, by South Korean researchers at Seoul National University where earlier, human embryos had been cloned and stem cells extracted. The surrogate mother of this cloned dog was a yellow Labrador retriever. One hundred and twenty three dogs were used as both egg donors and surrogate mothers, and from over 1,000 prepared eggs or ova each containing a skin cell from a dog's ear, three pregnancies resulted, one ending in a miscarriage, one resulting in a pup that died soon after birth from respiratory failure, and the third a viable clone of a male Afghan hound. Some bioethicists fear that the cloning of man's best friend is the final stepping stone to eventual public acceptance of human cloning.

Cloning entails taking a single cell from an animal and placing the cell inside the egg case or ovum taken from another animal of the same species that has been emptied of its contents. After a procedure that activates the cell to begin to divide, the ovum containing the cloning cell is placed in the uterus of a hormonally receptive surrogate animal. Because of low success rates in getting the cloned cells to implant into the uterine wall, and because the placenta and embryo may not develop normally, several ova containing the clone cells may be put into the surrogate animal's uterus at the same time.

People taking a beloved dog or cat to the veterinarian for a routine health check will have a few cells removed, quickly frozen, and shipped for storage at a Pet Cloning Center. A processing and storage fee will be charged, and when the owners want their companion animals to be cloned, the Center will begin the process after a substantial down payment has been made, or full payment has been provided. Before this new biotechnology is perfected and large-scale operations set up with hundreds, possibly thousands, of caged and hormonally manipulated female dogs and cats serving as ova donors, and others being the recipients of ova containing the to-be-cloned pets' cells, the cost will probably be in the six-figure range for some time before mass-production follows mass-demand.

But there are many concerns other than financial:

The cloned dogs will not be exact replicas of peoples' beloved animal companions, and many clones will probably be spontaneously aborted, or have to be destroyed because of various birth defects. Abnormalities may also develop later in life. Clones of other species often have abnormal internal organs, neurological and immunological problems, and may be abnormally large at birth due to a defective growth-regulating gene function. What about the origins, quality of life and future of the thousands of caged female dogs who will be exploited by the pet cloning industry, and the procedural risks to their health and overall welfare? Do the ends justify the means? There is no evident benefit to the animals themselves.

Why not adopt from an animal shelter a dog or puppy who looks like the one you miss or might be passing on soon, who needs a good home; or donate money, equivalent to what it would cost to produce one clone, toward improving the welfare of hundreds, even thousands of dogs, and other animals in communities around the world?

What are these ends anyway? Certainly there is a commercial end that is potentially lucrative, given the right market promotion and endorsements by professionals and celebrities.

But is there real human benefit in making a clone of one's beloved canine companion? Or is it mere pandering to a misguided sentimentalism? Because of the close emotional bond between humans and their animal companions, the pet cloning business I see as an unethical exploitation of the bond for pecuniary ends. Exact replicas of peoples' dogs cannot be guaranteed, and will not likely be created because an identical environment during embryonic and postnatal development cannot be achieved. All clones may, at the time of birth, be of the same chronological age as the age of the cells taken from the to-be cloned animals. So if a cell is taken from a six-year-old dog, because of the aging "clock," the clone may already be aged by six years at the time it is born.

From various religious and spiritual perspectives and beliefs, cloning violates the sanctity of life and the integrity of divine or natural creative processes. It is problematic from the point of view of reincarnation, or transmigration of the soul. From a Buddhist perspective, the consciousness incarnate in the body of the clone, or the consciousnesses in the bodies of many clones from the same original animal, are all going to be different from the original donor.

It is not inconceivable that dog clones might also be created initially on an experimental basis, and used to provide spare parts such as kidneys, hearts, hips, and knees for ailing dogs. Research laboratories may also use cloning to quickly develop identical sets of dogs and other animals for biomedical research. Some sets and lines of clones having the same genetically engineered anomalies to serve as high fidelity models of various human diseases may be created and marketed to develop new and profitable drugs to treat these conditions in humans and other animals.

The bioethics and medical validity of these developments need to be examined. And pet owners who put out the money to have their animal companions cloned may want to think twice, since they may well be giving this new cloning business not only a financial jump start, but also the socio-political credibility that it needs in order to gain widespread public acceptance, and a market for human cloning and for other biologically anomalous and ethically dubious products and processes.

The fact that a venture capitalist made a grant of $2.3 million and hired an agent to find a university biotech Laboratory already in the cloning business to clone his dog Missy (visit www.missyplicity.com) and the subsequent public relations and media promotion of this project, points to another agenda: The cloning of pets may be a ploy to promote human cloning. If the cloning of pets becomes a reality, the public will become desensitized to the issue of cloning and more likely to eventually accept a highly lucrative biotechnology for childless couples and rich and selfish singles for the cloning of complete human beings, and of partial human beings (such as anencephalics or headless clones) as a source of replacement tissues and organ parts.

The Philosophy Department at Texas A&M University, where the Missyplicity Project was started in another department before being spun off into a private company "Genetics, Savings and Clone," developed a set of 'bioethical guidelines' based on the ethical principle of what they call axiomatic anthropocentrism. This strategy was clearly designed to deflect public criticism and concern over the morality and animal welfare aspects of the Project. Axiomatic anthropocentrism essentially means whatever is good for a person is ethically acceptable. Anthropocentrism, human centeredness, is an outmoded worldview or paradigm that many advocates of animal rights and environmental protection see as the root cause of untold animal suffering and ecological devastation over the millennia.

Several female dogs were put up for adoption on the web site, one of the company's 'bioethical principles' being that regardless of the source through which dogs are obtained for use as egg donors or surrogate mothers, (from animal shelters, breeding, farms, etc.), at the completion of their role in the Missyplicity Project, all dogs shall be placed in loving homes. No funds shall be expended for dogs raised under inhumane conditions, such as puppy mills.

The Missyplicity Project included several goals in addition to the cloning of Missy that were published on the web site. These included dozens, perhaps hundreds, of scientific papers on canine reproductive physiology; enhanced reproduction and repopulation of endangered wild canids; plans to develop improved canine contraceptive and sterilization methods as a way of preventing the millions of unwanted dogs who are euthanized in America every year; to clone exceptional dogs of high societal value, especially search-and-rescue dogs; and develop low-cost commercial dog-cloning services for the general public.

These goals gave the Project the kind of credibility that a gullible public and organizations and professionals with a limited grasp of the inherent limitations and harmful consequences of cloning, would readily accept. Ethical concerns and the questions concerning the validity and relevance of applying cloning biotechnology to wildlife conservation, to dog overpopulation, and to the propagation of high performance dogs were cleverly deflected by these promissory goals.

Genetic Savings and Clone, the commercial spin-off from the Missyplicity Project at Texas A&M University, launched 'Operation CopyCat' in 2000. The company estimated that the price for cloning a cat or dog would drop to $25,000 within three years. They never succeeded in cloning a dog, and eventually went out of business, but a northern California biotech company, BioArts International, created several cloned cats for sale at $ 50,000 each, that turned out to be a commercial flop.

Undaunted, BioArts linked with the disgraced cloning scientist Hwang Woo Suk who had succeeded in cloning dogs in Korea, in an effort to market cloned dogs in the US in 2008 (Woo Suk was still under indictment for embezzling research funds in Korea, and for violating ethics laws in the course of acquiring hundreds of eggs from women for his cloning research, when his business association with BioArts International was made). BioArts International set up a public auction to clone five dogs for willing customers, with bids starting at $100,000! In another publicity stunt, this company offered owners a free chance to have their dogs cloned, and chose the German shepherd rescue dog who worked in the rubble of the 9/11 terrorist attack at the World Trade Center in new York city, as the 'most clone-worthy canine.'

A-8. Behavioral Problems & Drug Solutions: A Last Resort

A variety of psychotropic drugs have proven to be beneficial for treating people with various emotional and behavioral problems, such as anxiety, depression, and obsessive-compulsive disorders. Veterinarians are discovering that these drugs can help in treating similar problems in dogs. These clinical findings support my contention that the inner world of dogs, their consciousness and emotionality, must be similar in many ways to ours, otherwise these psychotropic drugs would not result in similar clinical improvement in dogs as in human patients.

Veterinarians are well advised to use behavioral-modification techniques like reward training, desensitization, changing the dog's environment, and evaluating the dog-human relationships in the home before prescribing these kinds of drugs. Some have potentially harmful side effects. Then there is the ethical issue of giving drugs to dogs to help them cope with a way of life — like being left alone (often in a crate) for many hours during the work week, to which no animal should be subject. Turning a dog into a chemically-dependent zombie is ethically untenable.

The benefits of these mind (brain-chemistry) and behavior-altering drugs to dogs are being documented in the veterinary literature. Before the advent of these new drugs, many dogs would suffer years of distress (and their owners too), or be euthanized.

Fluoxetine (Dista's Prozac) has helped many dogs suffering from obsessive-compulsive disorders, including compulsive licking, pacing, tail-chasing, and self-mutilation. Selegiline (Pfizer's Anipryl) is now being prescribed for old dogs suffering from the "old dog's disease" of disorientation and anxiety called cognitive dysfunction syndrome. Amitriptylene (Zeneca's Elevil) is one of several medications that can help dogs showing dominance aggression, coupled with underlying anxiety. Buspirone (Bristol-Myers Squibb's BuSpar) and Clomipramine (Novartis' Clomicalm) have proven beneficial to dogs suffering from fear-related aggression.

One of the most common emotional disorders to afflict dogs today is separation anxiety. If behavior-modification techniques, and providing another dog as a companion or an open crate as a safe "den" do not work, the treatment with any of the above drugs, including Eli Lilly's Reconcile (that is the same as Prozac but is beef-flavored), or with Imipramine (Novartis' Tofranil) or Alprazolam (Pharmacia and Upjohns' Xanax) can provide significant relief, emotionally or symptomatically, for the dog, which will help the distraught owners feel better as well.

I find it ethically questionable to drug a dog who is suffering from boredom and loneliness and becomes a house-wrecker. Wherever possible, dogs' basic needs should be met and their environments changed for their benefit rather than changing their brain chemistry to help them cope with and adapt to a relatively deprived existence. Is it more ethical to selectively breed them to better adapt to such conditions? Or would they then become "virtual dogs," dispirited facsimiles of the once real, that our children may never know, respect and cherish, with no remnant of the wild that we recognized in their original presence?

Many behavioral and emotional problems in dogs have a complex genesis, including the animal's genetic background and basic temperament, the dog's rearing history and experiences earlier in life, and current factors in the dog's immediate environment and family relations, including other animals as well as people in the home.

The judicious use of psychotropic drugs, with careful monitoring and individual dose-adjustments is appropriate, I believe, but only as a last resort for those conditions when behavioral counseling and modification procedures have failed. Often the dogs can be slowly weaned off these drugs and, in the process, they seem to learn to cope better with the conditions or stimuli that caused their behavioral disturbance in the first place.

The worst side-effect of some psychotropic drugs (other than dependence, liver damage and paradoxical reactions), which lead me to caution against over-prescribing, are disturbing consequences that may be hard to detect in the animal, but which humans report when on similar drugs. These may include disorientation, increased feelings of vulnerability, anxiety or depression, fatigue, loss of appetite, and disturbed sleep patterns.

Another often overlooked factor that can affect behavior is diet. Nutritionists are beginning to discover how dietary habits cannot only affect the immune system and other vital body functions, but also influence behavior, emotions, and cognitive (learning) abilities in humans. Recent work by a team of veterinarians at Tuft's University School of Veterinary Medicine, Boston, has revealed that for dogs showing territorial aggression, their aggressive behavior was lowered when they were fed a low protein diet supplemented with tryptophan (10 mg/kg per meal, twice daily). Dogs showing dominance aggression were less aggressive when fed low or high protein diets supplemented with tryptophan, compared to when they were fed a high protein diet without the extra tryptophan. These different diets had no appreciable effect on hyperactive dogs.

While a dietary approach to treating some dog behavior problems is relatively new, the health benefits of good nutrition have been long recognized. Artificial coloring agents, preservatives and other ingredients like wheat and various glutens in many manufactured foods may affect brain and behavior, so a whole-food, biologically appropriate diet may be helpful. Many veterinarians prescribe herbal and nutraceutical supplements for companion animals with behavioral and emotional problems including Valerian, Passion flower, Hops, Lavender, Kava Kava, Chamomile, and Melatonin.

The need for companionship for a dog alone at home all day should also be considered, another compatible dog, or a cat or two being the most natural remedy, and negating the need for psychotropic drugs to help an animal cope with loneliness and a deprived, unstimulating environment.

A-9. Pharmaceutical Cruelty Down Factory Pig Farm

The documentation given in this article should put all on notice, including pet owners whose pets may be eating pet foods containing pork byproducts. A drug called PAYLEAN is now being used widely by the pig industry. The FDA has also recently approved its use in cattle (See Figures 9-1-3, p. 78).

Pigs are curious, intelligent, playful, and sociable creatures, tending to be more cautious than placid like cows, but they can be very aggressive when feeling threatened. Dosing them with Paylean, a beta-adrenoreceptor agonist, is the cruelest thing to do to the pig's psyche—or to any creature's state of mind and sense of well-being. This drug destabilizes the pig's physiological and psychological homeostasis and subjective sense of well-being, evident in their heightened, chronic states of irritability, agitation, flightiness, and aggressiveness. This new drug, given to make them lean-muscled when fed on a sickening diet of corn and soy (publicly subsidized no less), makes their lives in crowded pens hideously stressful by super-stimulating their adrenal-systems. This means more fear and fighting until the stressed survivors are heavy enough to go out of the factory shed to slaughter. Their increased muscle mass makes normal movements difficult, and creates difficulties loading them for transport to slaughter, during which time they bruise easily and suffer great stress.

This is pharmacological cruelty of the first order—chemical torture, simply for profit, certainly not for public health (making pigs more lean). Such highly-wound up, physiologically challenged and psychologically disturbed creatures will have impaired immune function, increasing their susceptibility to diseases. Antibiotics are used by the thousands of pounds to keep the pigs alive and eating, making industrial pig factories the new epicenters for zoonotic diseases—bacterial and viral diseases transmitted to people.

Since animal studies show that only about 80 percent of this drug is excreted in the pigs' feces and urine, that means twenty percent of the drug ractopamine hydrochloride, marketed as Paylean, remains in the pigs' body, including parts people consume. It is my considered opinion that residues of this 'speed'-like drug in pork products raise the question of significant health risks to a vulnerable segment of the population, especially those on adrenal, autonomic, neuro-endocrine and immune-system affecting prescription drugs. Animal studies that have been conducted on the effects of this drug on rats, dogs, and monkeys, as well as pigs, give no such guarantee, to my knowledge, of unconditional consumer safety.

Paylean, approved a decade ago by the Federal government for pig producers to use, is a product of Elanco technology, a company owned by Eli Lilly. To some cultures and way of thinking, this is a great product. For me it is an abomination; a shameful reflection of a species of depraved existence rather than exalted communion with other sentient beings as I have experienced seeing how piglets play, hogs wallow, and sows go ballistic defending their young from my needle and knife. But never would I have dreamed, as a young vet student working on Yorkshire pig farms fifty years ago, that there would come a time when pigs would be drugged just for profit, and that there could ever be of such widespread and insidious animal exploitation and evident, yet sanctioned cruelty and suffering.

This new administration should recall the Farm Bill and cut out all public subsidies associated with all livestock and poultry production practices that are not organically certified and humane. All consumers should avoid all pork products that do not clearly have a USDA certified "Antibiotic & Paylean free" label if they do consume pork, ham, sausage or bacon. It should be noted that 15 people in China were arrested recently by their government for selling this drug illegally to pig farmers, and that while there are no restrictions for its use in Canada, all pork products exported to the European Union countries must be from pigs never given this outrageously misapplied pharmaceutical product.

A-10. Mammon Versus Civil Society

The two world views that reflect the conflict of values between the rights and interests of civil society and of the corporate imperialists are as irreconcilable as they are ancient. It is the conflict between domination, expropriation and exploitation, versus cooperation, participation, and conservation. This is no better illustrated today than by the imposition of genetically engineered (GE) seeds and crops on states and countries where civil society opposition is overruled by government collaboration with the rising global biotechnocracy.

This technocracy, following the dictum of Henry Kissinger, former US Secretary of State who said "If you want to control the people, control the food," now seeks control through the patent monopoly of seed, conveniently ignoring the genetic contamination of conventional and organic crops by its GE plants. The health, safety, and nutritional value of GE crops and foods was presumed, but never proven. The control motivation is for world-market penetration and domination in the service of mammon—profits and power. Social and other external costs and risks are of no consequence, the entire transnational business enterprise being amoral, 'science-based', and devoid of any bioethical evaluation. It is insulated by aligned governments and organizations and agencies like the World Trade Organization, and FAO/WHO Codex Alimentarius, from public accountability and responsibility for harms done including its significant contribution to climate change with its primary production of feed for livestock and poultry, and now for biofuels.

Their seeds are primarily for commodity crops not grown to feed people directly and locally, making a few very rich, while more go hungry as more still, along with their pets, become sick consuming manufactured, highly processed convenience, junk, and fast-foods that are served widely in public schools.

What the mother eats during pregnancy creates an imprint on the developing child, so called nutritional epigenetics, that can mean chronic health problems are passed on from generation to generation. Now there are food riots around the world as prices rise because of climate change-related crop failures, and basic food crops and arable land being used to produce ecologically damaging biofuels.

Other less visible seeds are sown by the hands of the antidisestablishmentarians that blossom in the educational system especially, leading to public ignorance, indifference, consumerism, false trust and hope, as well as obedience and conformity. But learned helplessness, frustration, and the emptiness of modern existence devoid of values other than material, are taking their toll on mental health, leading to depression, violence and a host of socio-emotional disorders aggravated by spiritual poverty as much as by economic poverty. Diet plays a significant role in the genesis of these disorders. The old opiates of alcohol and religion, and the new opiates of illegal drugs and widely prescribed psychotropic drugs given even to kindergarten children, do little to ameliorate such cultural 'dis-ease.'

The looming specters of world hunger and the emerging health care crisis in industrialized, developed nations are being exacerbated rather than alleviated by this agribusiness sector of the food, drug and military-industrial complex. The declining health and increasing public health costs in developed countries correlate with low incomes and socio-economic stress, the more educated and affluent sectors having fewer stress and diet-related health problems that are becoming epidemic in lower social strata. This social gradient of disease for the underprivileged means elevated blood cortisol levels, impaired immune systems with lowered resistance to infections, diabetes, obesity, arteriosclerosis, high blood pressure, stroke, and heart attacks, chronic diseases such as osteoarthritis and cancer, and premature ageing. These and other diseases of modern civilization are anthropogenic; man made in the service of mammon. The rich ride the unstoppable juggernaut they call 'progress' that will only be derailed when civil society gains control, first in the realm of food and nutrition, the cornerstones of health for generations to come.

Corporate imperialism, sustained by the industrial-military complex of western capitalism, brainwashes citizens into believing that they live in a democracy rather than a technocracy. War and 'preemptive strikes' are justified in the name of peace and freedom. Such Orwellian newspeak and double-think reached the point in the Bush administration that any threats to corporate interests were seen as a threat to the economy and to national security. Animal rights activists, environmentalists and conservationists were identified as potential terrorist groups.

Now, sound science and reason are being trumped, according to science historians Naomi Oreskes and Eric M. Conway (See their book *Merchants of Doubt*, Bloomsbury Press, 2010) by a handful of scientists (backed by big corporations with their high-paid government lobbyists and well funded 'think tank' institutions like the Hastings, Heartland and Cato Institutes), to spread doubt and disinformation on a host of public health and environmental issues in order to prevent or delay much needed government regulations especially with regard to climate change, pesticides, food safety and even the risks of tobacco smoke. Biased media reporting, under the dictum of giving all sides or points of view equal exposure, serves only to confuse the public and further delay responsible government action. There are no sides to truth when it is based on sound science and objective documentation. But facts can be fabricated, scientific data manipulated and risks discounted to serve those vested interests of oligopolies whose agenda is not the public good but the protection of corporate hegemony.

We will never stop this juggernaut until civil society is unified by visionary leaders who have no vested interest in preserving the status quo where the common good is sacrificed for the corporate good. The possibility of a sustainable economy and a more viable future has been put in grave jeopardy by the corrupted values and short-term profit motives (basically greed) of the power elite.

The ignoble heroics of colonialism and empire building for God, King, and Country, one of the insanities of the past three centuries, has evolved into the insanity of transnational corporate imperialism. Under the neo-liberal banner of 'free' rather than fair trade, and in the wake of missionary zeal, military might, and political and market manipulation and control, the cancerous monoculture of mammon has spread globally. This consumption-driven juggernaut leaves in its wake decimated communities and cultures and devastated environments devoid of wildlife and natural resources, from fresh water and good topsoil to clean air and healthy forests and other natural ecosystems upon which our health and basic economy depend.

The quickening of climate change, ecocide, plant and animal species and community extinctions, and the loss of law and order, ethics and compassion, call for a full examination of what we are living for and how we all might live less consumptively and harmfully.

Surely the value of our lives is ultimately in how much is given rather than taken. Where there is compassion, conscience, and concern there is kinship, justice, and hope. Where there is none of these, there is no civilization, only the anarchism of materialism, consumerism and egotism; and inhumanity and insanity. As human history informs, there will always be war and poverty, famine and pestilence when ego comes before eco; self before other.

Every civilization that broke this covenant of compassionate stewardship with the natural world either became extinct or endured into the present as dysfunctional, strife-torn cultures and nation states. Ours in the West is no different, as we bear witness to the tragic consequences of egotism, chauvinism, and anthropocentrism that are outmoded modes of being. We must choose to either evolve as a human, and therefore humane, species, or perish under our collective inhumanity toward animals, nature and our own species.

Many who lament how medical, technological and other 'advances' for the betterment of society so often have unanticipated harmful consequences, attribute such nemesis to a lack of prescience or foresight and vision. Consequential considerations are part of the bioethical evaluation of any new medical or other products and services. These considerations include more than safety and effectiveness, and short and narrowly focused risk-benefit determinations. Economic, ecological, environmental, social and often political, corporate and legal considerations are often paramount. In market-economic terms these are the 'externalities' or hidden costs of collateral damage. Also one's professional and personal beliefs, values and motives, from the perspectives of cultural relativity, historical precedents and the experiences and concerns of others together may give us the degree of prescience coupled with the precautionary principle to better insure human creativity does more good than harm.

We are losing all sense and evidence of our humanity at an alarming rate. But belief and circumstance need not dictate our fate if we adhere to the cardinal virtues of honesty, humility, and respect for all life. To believe and act otherwise is the nemesis of humanity. To show compassion toward the perpetrators of violence as well as to the victims calls for the tempering of moral outrage, condemnation, and retaliation, empathy being the compass for ethical direction.

The manifest reality of this living universe is as terrifying as it is awe inspiring in its beauty, intelligent design, and creative organization. Yet before we have even begun to understand the nature of reality—the laws of Nature, of quantum fields and of genetic processes—in order to learn the art of living and the science of health, we plunder and desecrate. We live in a time and culture where nonliving entities like corporations, but not living entities like trees and oceans, have legal standing. The more that we distance ourselves from, and destroy the last of the wild, the less the natural world can serve as a referential for the human spirit and for our ethical and empathic sensibilities, without which we are no longer human. To have no feeling for the harpooned whale, the chained elephant, the caged tiger and the crated sow is to become less than human.

The choice between egocentrism or eco-centrism as modes of being and consciousness has been made—welcome to the modern age!

But in reality we have no choice if we are to evolve and become givers rather than takers, more fully human, humane, because being altruistic is enlightened self-interest. When we take care of the Earth the Earth will take care of us. Earth First!

From this holistic view, the first order of business is to educate the populace to support government subsidized, organic food producers as one of the cornerstones of public health and environmental restoration. Home economics needs to be reinstated as part of the high school curriculum as it was a generation ago, teaching students the basics of nutrition, food selection, preparation and storage; and inspiring self-reliance in the kitchen and enabling informed choices to be made in the marketplace. Inculcating the values of the Three Rs—repair, reuse, recycle—is surely the way to a more sustainable future and the antidote to the waste and ruin of global consumerism that ultimately consumes itself.

END NOTES & CITATIONS

Chapter 4
For Further Reading:
Fox, Michael W. (1997) *Eating with Conscience: The Bioethics of Food*.
    Troutdale, OR: New Sage Press.
Hamaker, John D. and Donald A. Weaver (1982) *Survival of Civilization*.
    Seymour, MO: Hamaker-Weaver Publishers.
Israel, Richard (1991) *Natural Pharmacy Product Guide*. Garden City, NJ:
    Avery.

Chapter 5
Badgley, C., et al, (2007) Organic agriculture and the global food supply.
    Renewable Agriculture and Food Systems, 22:86-108.
Balcome, J. (2006) *Pleasurable Kingdom: Animals and the Nature of Feeling Good*.
    New York, Macmillan.
Bekoff, M. (2007) *The Emotional Lives of Animals*. Novato CA, New World
    Library.
Berry, T. (1988) *The Dream of the Earth*. San Francisco, CA, Sierra Books.
Campbell, T.C. (2005) *The China Study: The Most Comprehensive Study of
    Nutrition Conducted, and the Startling Implication for Diet, Weight-loss and
    Long-term Health*. Dallas TX Bell Bella Books.
Cooper, J., Leifert, C., and Niggily, U., (eds) (2007) *Handbook of Organic Food
    Safety and Quality*. Cambridge, UK Woodhead Pub Inc.
Diamond, J. (2005) *Collapse: How Societies Choose to Fail or Succeed*. New York,
    Penguin Books.
Domingo, J.L. (2007) Toxicity Studies of Genetically Modified Plants: A
    Review of Published Literature. *Critical Reviews in Food Science and
    Nutrition* 47:721-733.
Einstein, A. (1954) *Ideas and Opinions*. Carl Seelig (ed), New York, Crown
    Publishing.
Fox, M. W. (1995) Veterinary bioethics: ecoveterinary and ethnoveterinary
    perspectives. *Vet. Res. Commun.* 19: 9-15.
_____ (1997) *Eating With Conscience: The Bioethics of Food*. Troutdale,

OR. New Sage Press.

_____ (1998) *Veterinary Bioethics in Complementary and Alternative Medicine: Principles and Practice.* A.M. Schoen and S.G. Wynn (eds). St Louis MO, Mosby.

_____ (2001) *Bringing Life to Ethics: Global Bioethics for a Humane Society.* Albany, NY, State University of New York Press.

_____ (2004) *Killer Foods: What Scientists Do To Make Better Is Not Always Best.* Guilford CT, The Lyons Press.

_____ (2006) Principles of veterinary bioethics *JAVMA* 229, 666-667.

Goodland, R. (1997) Environmental Sustainability in Agriculture: Diet Matters. *Ecological Economics* 23: 189-200.

Hu, F. B., and Willett, W.C. (1998) *The Relationship Between Consumption of Animal Products (Beef, Pork, Poultry, Eggs, Fish and Dairy Products) and Risk of Chronic Disease: a Critical Review. Report for the World Bank.* Cambridge, MA, Harvard School of Public Health.

Imhoff, D., and Baumgartner, J. A. (eds) (2006) *Farming and the Fate of Wildlife.* Healdsburg, CA, Watershed Media.

Korten, D. (1995) *The Tyranny of the Global Economy.* West Hartford, CT

Margulis, L (1998) *The Symbiotic Planet: A New Look at Evolution.* New York, Basic Books.

McMillan, F.D. (ed), (2005) *Mental Health and Well-Being in Animals.* Blackwell, Ames Iowa.

Potter, V.R., (1971) *Bioethics: Bridge to the Future.* Englewood Cliffs, NJ, Prentice Hall.

Rollin, B. E. (2006) *An Introduction to veterinary Medical Ethics: Theory and Cases.* Ames, Iowa, State University Press.

Schweitzer, A. (1965) *The Teaching of Reverence for Life.* New York, Holt, Rinehart and Winston.

Webster, J. (2005) Limping Towards Eden. London, Blackwell.

Wilson, A.K., Latham, J.R., and Steinbrecher, R.A.(2006) Transformation-induced mutations in transgenic plants: Analysis and biosafety implications. *Biotechnology and Genetic Engineering Reviews*, 23, p 209-226.

Steinfeld, H.P., Gerber, T., Wassenaar, V., et al (2006) *Livestock's Long Shadow: Environmental Issues and Options.* Rome. Food and Agriculture Organization.

Chapter 6

A. Fraser (1991) p. 932 in *Merck Veterinary Manual.* Rahway, NJ: Merck & Co. 1978, Minnesota, University of Minnesota Press.

For example see C. Schwabe *Veterinary Medicine and Human Health* 3rd Ed. (1984), Baltimore, Williams and Wilkins.

For extensive documentation see N.J. Temple and D.P. Burkitt (1994) *Western Diseases: Their Dietary Prevention and Reversibility*, Totowa, New Jersey, Humana Press.

For example, see *Ethnoveterinary Medicine in Asia*, International Institute for Rural Reconstruction, Y.C. James Yen Center, Silang Phillipines (1995) and C.M. McCorkle et al. (eds), Ethnoveterinary Research and Development, London, Intermediate Technology Publications (in Press).

See C.M. McCorkle, *Intersectoral Health care Delivery in Alternative Perspectives on Health: An Ecological Approach*, J. Chesworth (ed.), Thousand Oaks, California, Sage Publications. (1995).

See Fox, M.W., (1992), *The Place of Farm Animals in Humane Sustainable Agriculture*, Washington, D.C., The Humane Society of the United States, and C.M. McCorkle (ed.), (1992), *Plants, Animals and People: Agropastoral Systems Research*, Boulder, CO, Westview Press. Bayer, W. Waters-Bayer, A. (1989), Crop-livestock Interactions for Sustainable Agriculture, Gatekeeper Series Briefing Paper, Sustainable Agriculture Programme, London, International Institute for Environment and Development. Bostid/NRC, (1991), Microlivestock, Little-known Small Animals with a Promising Economic Future, Washington, D.C., National Academy Press for the Board on Science and Technology for International Development, the National Research Council.

See M.W. Fox (1986) *Laboratory Animal Husbandry: Ethology, Welfare and Experimental Variables*, Albany, New York, State University of New York Press.

For an excellent text for animal caretakers, see R. Kilgour and C. Dalton (1984), *Livestock Behavior: A Practical Guide*, Boulder, CO, Westview Press.

For a comprehensive review of this fascinating and important aspect of the human-animal bond, see P.H. Hemsworth, et al. (1993) The human-animal relationship in agriculture and its consequences for the animal. *Animal Welfare* (Universities Federation for Animal Welfare) 2:33-51.

For details, see J.F. Seabrook (1994) the effect of production systems on the behavior and attitudes of stockpersons. pp. 252-8 in Proc. 4th Zodiac Symposium. *Biological Basis of Sustainable Animal Production.* EAAP. Publ.. No. 67. Waneningen, the Netherlands.

See M.W. Fox (2004) *Killer Foods: When Scientists Manipulate Genes, Better is Not Always Best.* Guilford CT. The Lyons Press.

For a comprehensive review, see A.T.B. Edney (1992) Companion animals and human health. *Veterinary Record,* April 4, p. 285-87.

Chapter 7

For more details on this modern food crisis and its adverse effects on companion animals, see *Not Fit For a Dog: The Truth About Manufactured Dog And Cat Food* by veterinarians Drs. M.W. Fox, E. Hodgkins, and M. E. Smart, published in 2008 by Quill Driver Books, Sanger, CA.

Organically certified foods of both animal and plant origin contain more essential nutrients, notably antioxidants, than conventionally grown produce, and of course cause less environmental harms and are pesticide free. For documentation, see Cooper J, Leifert C, and Niggily U, (eds) *Handbook of Organic Food Safety and Quality.* Cambridge, UK, Woodhead Publ. Inc. 2007.

For evidence that organic farming methods can feed the hungry world, see Badgley C, et al, Organic agriculture and the global food supply. *Renewable Agriculture and Food Systems,* 22:86-108, 2007.

Campbell, T.C, *The China Study: The most comprehensive study of nutrition conducted, and the startling implication for diet, weight-loss and long-term health.* Dallas TX Bell Bella Books, 2005.

Fox, M.W. *Bringing Life to Ethics: Global Bioethics for a Humane Society.* Albany, NY. State University of New York Press, 2001.

News and Reports. Rats reveal risks of 'junk food' during pregnancy. *The Veterinary Record,* Aug 18, p 215, 2007.

Steinfeld, H, P. Gerber P, Wassenaer T, Castel V, Rosales M, and de Haan C, *Livestock's Long Shadow: Environmental Issues and Options.* United Nation's Food and Agriculture Organization, Washington, DC, 2006.

Chapter 8

1. Lazarou J, Pomeranz BH, Corey PN. Incidence of adverse drug reactions in hospitalized patients: a meta-analysis of prospective studies. *JAMA*.1998; 279:1200-1205.
2. Cox S, *Sick Planet: Corporate Food and Medicine*. Ann Arbor, MI, 2008.
3. Fox MW, Hodgkins HE, Smart M. *Not Fit For a Dog: The Truth About Manufactured Dog And Cat Food*. Sanger, CA QuillDriver Books 2008.
4. McMillan FD. (ed) *Mental Health and Well-Being in Animals*. Ames, Iowa, Blackwell, 2005.
5. Schoen AM, S.G. Wynn SG. (eds) *Complementary and Alternative Medicine: Principles in Practice*. St Louis, MO, Mosby, 1998.
6. Fox MW. (ed) *Abnormal Behavior in Animals*. Philadelphia, PA, W.B. Saunders, 1968.
7. Fox MW. *Integrative Development of Brain and Behavior in the Dog*. Chicago, IL, University of Chicago Press, 1971.
8. Darwin C. *The Descent of Man and Selection in Relation to Sex*. New York, J.A. Hill & Co., 1904.
9. Eiseley L. *The Unexpected Universe*. New York, Harcourt, Brace and World, 1964.

Chapter 9
Selected References & Resources

Badgley, C, et al, Organic agriculture and the global food supply. *Renewable Agriculture and Food Systems*, 22:86-108, 2007.
Berry, T, *The Dream of the Earth*, San Francisco, CA, Sierra Books, 1988.
Berry, W, *The Unsettling of America: Culture and Agriculture*, New York, Avon, 1978.
Campbell, TC, *The China Study: The most comprehensive study of nutrition conducted, and the startling implication for diet, weight-loss and long-term health*. Dallas TX Bell Bella Books, 2005.
Cherfas, J, and M. & J. Fanton, *The Seed Saver's Handbook*, Chichester, UK, Grover books, 1996. See also International Pant Genetic Resources Institute www.ipgri.cgiar.org
Cooper, J, Leifert C, and Niggily U, (eds) *Handbook of Organic Food Safety and Quality*, Cambridge, UK 2007.
Diamond, J., *Collapse: How Societies Choose to Fail or Succeed*. New York, Penguin Books, 2005.
Domingo, J.L., Toxicity Studies of Genetically Modified Plants: A Review of Published Literature, *Critical Reviews in Food Science and Nutrition*

47:721-733, 2007.

Emmons, H, *The Chemistry of Joy*, New York, Simon and Shuster, 2006.

Ewald, P.W, The Evolution of Virulence. *Scientific American*, April, p 86-93, 1993.

Fox MW, *Farm Animals: Husbandry, Behavior and Veterinary Practice*. Baltimore MD, 1984. *Agricide: The Hidden Farm and Food Crisis that Affects us All*. New York, Schocken books, 1988. *Eating With Conscience: The Bioethics of Food* Troutdale OR, New Sage Press. 1997. *Bringing Life to Ethics: Global Bioethics for a Humane Society*. Albany, NY State University of New York Press, 2001. *Killer Foods: What Scientists Do To Make Better Is Not Always Best*. Guilford CT The Lyons Press 2004.

Fukuoka M, *The Natural Way of Farming: The Theory and Practice of Green Philosophy*, New York, Japanese Publications Inc., 1985

Goodland R, Environmental Sustainability in Agriculture: Diet Matters. *Ecological Economics*, 23: 189-200, 1997.

Hu Frank B. and Walter C. Willett, *The Relationship Between Consumption of Animal Products (Beef, Pork, Poultry, Eggs, Fish and Dairy Products) and Risk of Chronic Disease: a Critical Review. Report for the World Bank.* Cambridge, MA, Harvard School of Public Health, 1998

Imhoff D, and Baumgartner J A, (eds) *Farming and the Fate of Wildlife,* Healdsburg, CA, Watershed Media, 2006.

Jackson D.L, and Jackson L..L, (eds) *The Farm as Natural Habitat: Reconnecting Food Systems With Ecosystems,* Washington DC, Island Press, 2002

Korten D, *The Tyranny of the Global Economy*, West Hartford, CT, 1995.

Nieman, H. et al, Transgenic farm animals, *Rev. sci. Off. int. Epiz*, 24:285-298.

Organic salvation down on the farm, *New Scientist*, 184: p 9, 2004.

Pimental, D, Houser J, Preiss E, et al Water reserves: agriculture, the environment and society; an assessment of the status of water resources. *Bioscience* 47: 97-106, 1997.

Robbins J, *The Food Revolution: How Your Diet Can Help Save Your Life and Our World*, Newburyport, MA, 2001.

Robinson J, *Pasture Perfect: The Far-Reaching Benefits of Choosing Meat, Eggs, and Dairy Products from Grass-Fed Animals*. Vashon, WA, Vashon Island Press, 2004.

Schlosser E, *Fast Food Nation: The Dark Side of the All American Meal*, Boston MA, Houghton Mifflin, 2001

Smith J. M, *Genetic Roulette: The Documented Health Risks of Genetically Engineered Foods*, and visit his website www.seedsofdeception.com.

Smith J.R., *Tree Crops: A Permanent Agriculture*, Washington DC, Island Press,

1950.

Sokoloff, J, *The Politics of Food*, San Francisco, CA Sierra Books, 1985.

Steinfeld, H.P, Gerber T, Wassenaar V, et al. *Livestock's Long Shadow: Environmental Issues and Options*. Rome. Food and Agriculture Organization, 2006.

United Nations Development Programme, *Urban Agriculture: Food, Jobs and Sustainable Cities*, New York, UNDP, 1996.

Williams, C, *The Environmental Threat to Human Intelligence* a study funded by Britain's Economic and Social Research Council in its Global Environmental Change Programme, April 24, 2000.

Wilson, A.K, J.R. Latham, and R.A. Steinbrecher, Transformation-induced mutations in transgenic plants: Analysis and biosafety implications. *Biotechnology and Genetic Engineering Reviews*, 23, p 209-226, 2006.

Chapter 10
References

Organically certified foods of both animal and plant origin contain more essential nutrients, notably antioxidants, than conventionally grown produce, and of course cause less environmental harms and are pesticide free. For documentation, see Cooper J, Leifert C, and Niggily U, (eds) *Handbook of Food Quality and Safety*, Cambridge, UK, Woodhead Publ. Inc. 2007.

Badgley C, et al, Organic agriculture and the global food supply. *Renewable Agriculture and Food Systems*, 22:86-108, 2007.

Benachour, N. H., Sipahutar, S. Moslemi, C. Gasnier, C. Travert and G. E. Séralini, Time- and Dose-Dependent Effects of Roundup on Human Embryonic and Placental Cells, *Archives of Environmental Contamination and Toxicology*, online: 4 May 2007.

Benbrook, C. "Genetically Engineered Crops and Pesticide Use in the United States: The First Nine Years"; *BioTech InfoNet, Technical Paper Number 7*, October 2004.

Campbell, KH, Alberio R, Choi I, Fisher P, Kelly RD, Lee JH, Maalouf W. Cloning: eight years after Dolly. *Reprod Domest Anim.* 40(4):256-68. 2005.

Campbell, T.C, *The China Study: The most comprehensive study of nutrition conducted, and the startling implication for diet, weight-loss and long-term health*. Dallas TX Bell Bella Books, 2005.

Chowdhury, E. H., Kuribara, H., Hino, A., Sultana, P., Mikami, O.,

Shimada, N., Guruge, K. S., Saito, M., and Nakajima, Y. Detection of corn intrinsic and recombinant DNA fragments Cry1Ab protein in the gastrointestinal contents of pigs fed genetically modified corn Bt11. *J. Anim. Sci.* 81:2546–2551.2003.

Danish Centre for Bioethics and Risk Assessment (CeBRA). The science and technology of farm animal cloning: a review of the state of the art of the science, the technology, the problems, and the possibilities. *Report from the project Cloning in Public.* 2005 http://sl.kvl.dk/cloninginpublic/indexfiler/CloninginPublicTechnicalReport.pdf.

Domingo, José L. 'Toxicity Studies of Genetically Modified Plants: A Review of the Published Literature. *Critical Reviews in Food Science and Nutrition*, 47:8, 721 – 733, 2007.

Dona, A., and I.S. Arvanitoyannis, Health Risks of Genetically Modified Foods. *Critical Reviews in Food Science and Nutrition.* 49: 164-175, 2009.

Ermakova, I, Genetically modified soy leads to the decrease of weight and high mortality of rat pups of the first generation. Preliminary studies, *Ecosinform* 1: 4–9. 2006 (in Russian).

Ermakova, I. Genetically modified soy affects posterity: Results of Russian scientists' studies. Available online at: http://www.geneticsafety.org/info.php?txt-id=19&nid=776. 2005.

Ewen, S. W. B., and Pusztai, A. (1999a) Effect of diets containing genetically modified potatoes expressing Galanthus nivalis lectin on rat small intestine. *Lancet* 354:1353–1354.

Fox, M.W., *Bringing Life to Ethics: Global Bioethics for a Humane Society.* Albany, NY State University of New York Press, 2001.

Fox, M.W., *Killer Foods: What Scientists Do To Make Better is not Always Best.* Gulford, CT, The Lyons Press, 2004.

Griffin, H. Briefing notes on Dolly. *Roslin Institute Press Notice PN97-03.* December12 www.roslin.ac.uk/downloads/12-12-97-bn.pdf. 1997.

Grosse-Hovest, L. Müller, S. Minoia, R. Brem, G. Cloned transgenic farm animals produce a bispecific antibody for T cell-mediated tumor cell killing. *Proc Natl Acad Sci USA.* 2004 May 4; 101(18): 6858–6863.

Gurian-Sherman, D. *Failure to Yield.* Evaluating the Performance of Genetically Engineered Crops. Union of Concerned Scientists Publications, Cambridge Mass. April, 2009. (on line www.ucsusa.org).

Han, YM, Kang YK, Koo DB, and Lee KK. Nuclear reprogramming of cloned embryos produced in vitro. *Theriogenology* 59(1):33-44. 2003.

Hill, JR, Roussel AJ, Cibelli JB, et al. Clinical and pathologic features of cloned transgenic calves and fetuses (13 case studies). *Theriogenology*

51(8):1451-65. 1999.

Hu, Frank B. and Walter C. Willett, *The Relationship Between Consumption of Animal Products (Beef, Pork, Poultry, Eggs, Fish and Dairy Products) and Risk of Chronic Disease: a Critical Review*. Report for the World Bank. Cambridge, MA, Harvard School of Public Health, 1998.

Houdebine, LM. Production of pharmaceutical proteins by transgenic animals. *Comp Immunol Microbiol Infect Dis*. 32(2):91-105.2009.

Humphray, SJ, Scott CE, Clark R, Marron B, Bender C, Camm N, Davis J, Jenks A, Noon A, Patel M, Sehra H, Yang F, Rogatcheva MB, Milan D, Chardon P, Rohrer G, Nonneman D, de Jong P, Meyers SN, Archibald A, Beever JE, Schook LB, Rogers J. A high utility integrated map of the pig genome. *Genome Biol*. 8(7):R139. 2007.

Kaiser, M. Assessing ethics and animal welfare in animal biotechnology for farm production. *Rev Sci Tech*. Apr;24(1):75-87.2005

Kind A, Schnieke A. Animal pharming, two decades on. *Transgenic Res*.17(6):1025-33.2008

Laible, G. Enhancing livestock through genetic engineering—recent advances and future prospects. *Comp Immunol Microbiol Infect Dis*. 32(2):123-37. 2009.

Lassen J, Gjerris M, Sandøe P. After Dolly—ethical limits to the use of biotechnology on farm animals. *Theriogenology*. 65(5):992-1004 2006.

Leeson, S. "The Effect of Glufosinate Resistant Corn on Growth of Male Broiler Chickens," Department of Animal and Poultry Sciences, University of Guelph, *Report No. A56379*, July 12, 1996.

Loi, P, Clinton M, Vackova I, et al. Placental abnormalities associated with post-natal mortality in sheep somatic cell clones. *Theriogenology* 65(6):1110-21. 2006.

Malatesta, M, B. Baldelli, S. Battistelli, C. Tiberi, E. Manuali, M. Biggiogera, *Nuclear Changes Induced in Hepatocytes after GM Diet are Reversible*. 7th Multinational Congress on Microscopy—European Extension: 267-268 2005.

Malatesta, M, M. Biggiogera, E. Manuali, M. B. L. Rocchi, B. Baldelli, G. Gazzanelli, Fine Structural Analyses of Pancreatic Acinar Cell Nuclei from Mice Fed on GM Soybean. *Eur J Histochem* 47: 385-388. 2003.

Niemann, H, Kues WA. Transgenic farm animals: an update. *Reprod Domest Anim*. Jul;43 Suppl 2:355-8. 2008.

Oliveri, T et al., *Temporary Depression of Transcription in Mouse Pre-implantion Embryos from Mice Fed on Genetically Modified Soybean*, 48th Symposium of the Society for Histochemistry, Lake Maggiore (Italy), September

7–10, 2006.

Petersen, B, Carnwath JW, Niemann H. The perspectives for porcine-to-human xenografts. *Comp Immunol Microbiol Infect Dis*. 32(2):91-105. 2009.

Pusztai, A., Bardocz, S., and Ewen, S. W. B.. Genetically Modified Foods: Potential Human Health Effects. In: *Food Safety: Contaminants and Toxins* (ed) D'Mello JPF CAB International, Wallingford Oxon, UK, pp 347–372. 2003.

Robl, JM, Wang Z, Kasinathan P, Kuroiwa Y. Transgenic animal production and animal biotechnology. *Theriogenology*. 67(1):127-33. 2007.

Sabikhi, L. Designer milk. *Adv Food Nutr Res*.53:161-98 2007.

Saeki, K., Matsumoto, K., Kinoshita, M., Suzuki, I., Tasaka, Y., Kano, K. et al. Functional expression of a Delta12 fatty acid desaturase gene from spinach in transgenic pigs. *Proc. Natl. Acad. Sci. USA* 101:6361–6366.2004.

Schubbert, R., Renz, D., Schmitz, B., and Doerfler, W. Foreign (M13) DNA ingested by mice reaches peripheral leukocytes, spleen, liver via the intestinal wall mucosa can be covalently linked to mouse DNA. *Proc. Natl. Acad. Sci. USA* 94:961–966. 1997.

Seralini, G. E., Cellier, D., and de Venomois, J. S. New analysis of a rat feeding study with a genetically modified maize reveals signs of hepatorenal toxicity. *Arch. Environ. Contam. Toxicol*. Mar 13; [Epub ahead of print]. 2007.

Smith, J. M, *Genetic Roulette: The Documented Health Risks of Genetically Engineered Foods*, and visit his website www.seedsofdeception.com.

Steinfeld, H, P. Gerber P, Wassenaer T, Castel V, Rosales M, and de Haan C, *Livestock's Long Shadow: Environmental issues and Options* United Nation's Food and Agriculture Organization, Washington, DC, 2006.

Traavik, T and J. Heinemann, Genetic Engineering and Omitted Health Research: Still No Answers to Ageing Questions, *TWN Biotechnology & Biosafety Series 7*, 2007.

Tudisco, R. et al, Genetically Modified Soya Bean in Rabbit Feeding: Detection of DNA Fragments and Evaluation of Metabolic Effects by Enzymatic Analysis. *Animal Science* 82:193–199 2006.

Vajta, G, Gjerris M. Science and technology of farm animal cloning: state of the art. *Anim Reprod Sci*. 92(3-4):211-30.2006.

Vecchio, L et al, "Ultrastructural Analysis of Testes from Mice Fed on Genetically Modified Soybean," *European Journal of Histochemistry*

48::449–454. 2004.

Whitelaw, CB, Lillico SG, King T. Production of transgenic farm animals by viral vector-mediated gene transfer. *Reprod Domest Anim*. 43 Suppl 2:355-8.2008.

Williams, C, *The Environmental Threat to Human Intelligence*. A study funded by Britain's Economic and Social Research Council in its Global Environmental Change Programme, April 24, 2000.

Wilson, A.K, J.R. Latham, R.A. Steinbrecher, 'Transformation-induced mutations in transgenic plants: Analysis and biosafety implications. *Biotechnology and Genetic Engineering Reviews*, 23: 209-226, 2006.

Examples of Recent Research on GE & Cloned Farmed Animals

Ahmed Fadiel, Ifeanyi Anidi and Kenneth D. Eichenbaum Farm animal genomics and informatics: an update *Nucleic Acids Research*, 33:6308-6318, 2005.

Baldassarre, H, Schirm M, Deslauriers J, Turcotte C, Bordignon V. Protein profile and alpha-lactalbumin concentration in the milk of standard and transgenic goats expressing recombinant human butyrylcholinesterase. *Transgenic Res*. 2009 Mar 19. [Epub ahead of print]

Bösze, Z, Baranyi M, Whitelaw CB. Producing recombinant human milk proteins in the milk of livestock species. *Adv Exp Med Biol*. 2008; 606:357-93.

Brevini, TA, Antonini S, Pennarossa G, Gandolfi F. Recent progress in embryonic stem cell research and its application in domestic species. *Reprod Domest Anim*. 2008 Jul;43 Suppl 2:193-9.

Devlin, RH, Sakhrani D, Tymchuk WE, Rise ML, Goh B. Domestication and growth hormone transgenesis cause similar changes in gene expression in Coho salmon (Oncorhynchus kisutch). *Proc Natl Acad Sci U S A*. 2009 Mar 3;106(9):3047-52.

Fletcher, CJ, Roberts CT, Hartwich KM, Walker SK, McMillen IC. Somatic cell nuclear transfer in the sheep induces placental defects that likely precede fetal demise. *Reproduction*. 2007 Jan;133(1):243-55.

Golding, MC, Long CR, Carmell MA, Hannon GJ, Westhusin ME. Suppression of prion protein in livestock by RNA interference. *Proc Natl Acad Sci U S A*. 2006 Apr 4;103(14):5285-90.

Kues WA, Schwinzer R, Wirth D, Verhoeyen E, Lemme E, Herrmann D, Barg-Kues B, Hauser H, Wonigeit K, Niemann H. Epigenetic silencing and tissue independent expression of a novel tetracycline inducible system in double-transgenic pigs. *FASEB J*. 2006

Jun;20(8):1200-2.

McEvoy, TG, Alink FM, Moreira VC, Watt RG, Powell KA. Embryo technologies and animal health - consequences for the animal following ovum pick-up, in vitro embryo production and somatic cell nuclear transfer. *Theriogenology*. 2006 Mar 15;65(5):926-42.

Ortegon, H, Betts DH, Lin L, Coppola G, Perrault SD, Blondin P, King WA. Genomic stability and physiological assessments of live offspring sired by a bull clone, Starbuck II. *Theriogenology*. 2007 Jan 1; 67(1):116-26.

Quillet, E, Dorson M, Le Guillou S, Benmansour A, Boudinot P. Wide range of susceptibility to rhabdoviruses in homozygous clones of rainbow trout. *Fish Shellfish Immunol*. 2007 May; 22(5):510-9.

Salamone, D, Barañao L, Santos C, Bussmann L, Artuso J, Werning C, Prync A, Carbonetto C, Dabsys S, Munar C, Salaberry R, Berra G, Berra I, Fernández N, Papouchado M, Foti M, Judewicz N, Mujica I, Muñoz L, Alvarez SF, González E, Zimmermann J, Criscuolo M, Melo C. High level expression of bioactive recombinant human growth hormone in the milk of a cloned transgenic cow. *J Biotechnol*. 2006 Jul 13;124 (2):469-72.

Wise, TG, Schafer DS, Lowenthal JW, Doran TJ. The use of RNAi and transgenics to develop viral disease resistant livestock. *Dev Biol* (Basel). 2008;132:377-82.

Chapter 11
GM Food Hazard References

Adams, N. R. (1995). Detection of the effects of phytoestrogens on sheep and cattle. *J. Anim. Sci*. 73:1509–1515.

Alinorm 03/34 Joint FAO/WHO Food Standard Programme. 2003. C. A. C.: *Appendix III: Guideline for the conduct of food safety assessment of foods derived from recombinant-DNA plants; Appendix IV: Annex on the assessment of possible allergenicity*.

Alliance for Biointegrity website: http://www.biointegrity.org biointegrity. org (1998), including Calgene FLAVR SAVRTM tomato report, pp. 1-604; *International Research and Development Corp. first test report*, pp. 1736–1738.

Conclusions of the expert panel regarding the safety of the FLAVR SAVRTM tomato, ENVIRON, Arlington VA, USA pp. 2355–2382; Four week oral (intubation) toxicity study in rats by IRDC, pp. 2895–3000.

Aronson, A. I., and Shai, Y. (2001). Why Bacillus thuringiensis insecticidal toxins are so effective: unique features of their mode of action. *FEMS Microbiol Lett.* 195:1–8.

Arvanitoyannis, I. S., Choreftaki, S., and Tserkezou, P. (2005). An update of EU legislation (Directives and Regulations) on food-related issues (Safety, Hygiene, Packaging, Technology, GMOs, Additives, Radiation, Labeling): presentation and comments. *International Journal of Food Science and Technology.* 40(10):1021–1112.

Arvanitoyannis, I. S. (2006). Genetically modified plants In: *Microbial Biotechnology in Agriculture and Aquaculture*, volume II. Ray RC ed., Science Publishers, US, p.478–479.

Bakke-McKellep, A. M., Koppang E. O., Gunnes, G., Senden, M., Hemre, G.-I., Landsverk, T., and Krogdahl, A.(2007). Histological, digestive, metabolic, hormonal and some immune factor responses in Atlantic salmon, Salmo salar L., fed genetically modified soybeans. *J. Fish Dis.* 30:65–79.

Bannon, G., Fu, T. J., Kimber, I., Hinton, D. M. (2003). Protein digestibility and relevance to allergenicity. Environ. *Health Perspect.* 111:1122–4.

Beever, D. E, and Kemp, F. (2000). Safety issues associated with the DNA in animal feed derived from genetically modified crops. A review of scientific and regulatory procedures. *Nutr. Abst. Revs.* 70:197–204.

Bernstein, J. A., Bernstein, I. L., Bucchini, L., Goldman, L. R., Hamilton, R. G., Lehrer, S., and Rubin, C. (2003). Clinical and laboratory investigation of allergy to genetically modified foods. Environ. *Health Perspect* 111:1114–

Betz, F. S., Hammond, B. G., and Fuchs, R. L. (2000). Safety and advantages of Bacillus thuringiensis-protected plants to control insect pests. *Reg. Toxicol. Pharmacol.* 32:156–173.

Burlingame, B. (2004). Fostering quality data in food composition databases: visions for the future. *J. Food Comp. Anal.* 17:251–258.

Cellini, F., Chesson, A., Colquhoun, I., Constable, A., Davies, H. V., Engel, K. H., Gatehouse, A. M. R., K"arenlampi, S., Kok, E. J., Leguay, J.-J., Lehesranta, S., Noteborn, H. P. J. M., Pedersen, J., and Smith, M. (2004). Unintended effects and their detection in genetically modified crops. *Food Chem. Toxicol.* 42:1089–125.

Chan, J. M., Stampfer, M. J., Giovannucci, E., Gann, P. H., Ma, J., Wilkinson, P., Hennekens, C. H., and Pollak, M. (1998). Plasma insulin-like growth factor-I and prostate cancer risk: a prospective study. *Science* 279:563–564.

Chen, Z.-L., Gu, H., Li, Y., Su, Y., Wu, P., Jiang, Z., Ming, X., Tian, J., Pan, N., and Qu, L.-J. (2003). Safety assessment for genetically modified sweet pepper and tomato. *Toxicology* 188:297–307.

Chowdhury, E. H., Kuribara, H., Hino, A., Sultana, P., Mikami, O., Shimada, N., Guruge, K. S., Saito, M., and Nakajima, Y. (2003). Detection of corn intrinsic and recombinant DNA fragments Cry1Ab protein in the gastrointestinal contents of pigs fed genetically modified corn Bt11. *J. Anim. Sci.*81:2546–2551.

Conner, A. J., and Jacobs, J. M. E. (1999). Genetic engineering of crops as potential source of genetic hazard in the human diet. *Mutat. Res.* 443:223– 234.

Conner, A. J., Glare, T. R., and Nap, J. P. (2003). The release of genetically modified crops into the environment: Part II. Overview of ecological risk assessment. *Plant J.* 33:19–46.

Crevel, R. W., Cooper, K. J, Poulsen, L. K., Hummelshoj, L., and Bindslev-Jensen, C. (2007). Lack of immunogenicity of ice structuring protein type III HPLC12 preparation administered by the oral route to human volunteers. *Food Chem. Toxicol.* 45:79–87.

Demont, M., and Tollens, E. (2004). First impact of biotechnology in the EU: Bt maize adoption in Spain. *An. Appl. Biol.* 145:197–207.

De Schrijver, A., Devos, Y., van den Bulcke, M., Cadot, P., De Loose, M., Reheul, D., and Sneyers, M. (2007). Risk assessment of GM stacked events obtained from crosses between GM events. *Trends in Food Science and Technology.* 18:101–109.

Devos, Y., Maeseele, P., Reheul, D., van Speybroek, L., and Dewaele, D. (2007).

Ethics in the societal debate on genetically modified organisms: a (re)quest for sense and sensibility. *Journal of Agricultural and Environmental Ethics.* 21(1):29–61.

Devos, Y., Reheul, D., De Waele, D., and van Speybroeck, L. (2006). The interplay between societal concerns and the regulatory frame on GM crops in the European Union. *Environ. Biosafety Res.* 5:127–149.

Doerfler, W., and Schubbert R. (1998). Uptake of foreign DNA from the environment: the gastro-intestinal tract the placenta as portals of entry. *Wien Klin. Wochenschr* 110:40–44.

Dohoo, I. R., DesC^oteaux, L., Leslie, K., Fredeen, A., Shewfelt, W., Preston, A., and Dowling, P. (2003). A meta-analysis review of the effects of recombinant bovine somatotropin 2. Effects on animal health, reproductive performance, and culling. *Can. J. Vet. Res.* 67:252–264.

Dunham, R. A., and Devlin, R. H. (1999). Comparison of traditional breading and transgenesis in farmed fish with implications for growth enhancement and fitness. *Transgenic animals in agriculture*. Ed. J. D. Muray, G. B. Anderson.

A. M. Oberbauer, and M. M. McGloughlin, Wallingford CAB International. pp. 209–229. EFSA (European Food Safety Authority). (2005). Guidance document of the scientific panel on genetically modified organisms for the risk assessment of genetically modified plants and derived food feed. *The EFSA Journal 2004*, 99:1–94.

EFSA. (2006). Opinion of the scientific panel on genetically modified organisms on a request from the Commission related to the notification (C/SE/96/3501) for the placing on the market of genetically modified potato EH92-527-1 with altered starch composition, for the cultivation and production of starch, under Part C of Directive 2001/18/EC from BASF Plant Science. *EFSA J*. 323:1–20.

Einspanier, R., Klotz, A., Kraft, J., Aulrich, K., Poser, R., Schwaegle, F., Jahreis, G., and Flachowsky, G. (2001). The fate of forage plant DNA in farm animals, a collaborative case-study investigating cattle and chicken fed recombinant plant material. *Eur. Food Res. Technol*. 212:129–134.

Eppard, P. J., White, T. C., Sorbet, R. H., Weiser, M. G., Cole, W. J., Hartnell, G. F., Hintz, R. L., Lanza, G. M., Vicini, J. L., and Collier, R. J. (1997). Effect of exogenous somatotropin on hematological variables of lactating cows and their offspring. *J. Dairy Sci*. 80:1582–91.

Epstein, S. S. (1996). Unlabeled milk from cows treated with biosynthetic growth hormones: a case of regulatory abdication. *Int. J. Health Serv*. 26:173–85.

Ermakova, I. (2005). *Genetically modified soy affects posterity: Results of Russian scientists' studies*. Available online at: http:/www.geneticsafety.org/info. php?txt-id=19&nid=776.

Ewen, S.W.B., and Pusztai, A. (1999a) Effect of diets containing genetically modified potatoes expressing Galanthus nivalis lectin on rat small intestine. *Lancet* 354:1353–1354.

Ewen, S.W.B., and Pusztai A. (1999b). Effects of diets containing genetically modified potatoes expressing Galanthus nivalis lectin on rat small intestine. *Lancet* 354:1727–1728.

Exadactylos, A., and Arvanitoyannis I. S. (2006). Aquaculture biotechnology for enhanced fish production for human consumption.

In: *Microbial Biotechnology in Agriculture and Aquaculture*, volume II. Ray RC ed., Science Publishers, US, p. 478–479.

FAO/WHO. (2001). *Evaluation of allergenicity of genetically modified foods*. Report of a Joint FAO/WHO Expert Consultation on Foods Derived from Biotechnology, 22-15 January 2001, Rome Italy. Available: Food and Agriculture Organisation of the United Nations, Rome. http:// www.fao.org /es/esn/allergygm.pdf

Fares, N. H., and El-Sayed, A. K. (1998). Fine structural changes in the ileum of mice fed on delta-endotoxin-treated potatoes and transgenic potatoes. *Natural Toxins* 6:219–233.

Flachowsky, G., Chesson, A., and Aulrich, K. (2005). Animal nutrition with feeds from genetically modified plants. *Arch. Anim. Nutr.* 59:1–40.

Germolec, D. R., Kimber, I., Goldman, L., and Selgrade. (2003). Key issues for the assessment of the allergenic potential of genetically modified foods: Breakout group reports. *Environ. Health Perspect* 11:1131–1139.

Halford, N. G., and Shewry, P. R. (2000). Genetically modified crops: methodology, benefits, regulation and public concerns. *Brit. Med. Bull.* 56:71.

Hammond, B. G., Vicini, J. L, Hartnell, G. F., Naylor, M. W., Knight, C. D., Robinson, E. H., Fuchs, R. L., and Padgette, S. R. (1996). The feeding value of soybeans fed to rats chicken catfish and dairy cattle is not altered by genetic incorporation of glyphosate tolerance. *J. Nutr.* 126:717–727.

Hansen, M., Halloran, J. M., Groth, III, E. G., and Lefferts, L. Y. (1997). *Potential public health impacts of the use of recombinant bovine somatotropin in dairy production*. Prepared for a scientific review by the Joint Expert Committee on Food Additives.

Hill, R. H. Jr., Caudill, S. P., Philen, R. M., Bailey, S. L., Flanders, W. D., Driskell, W. J. et al. (1993). Contaminants in L-tryptophan associated with eosinophilia myalgia syndrome. *Arch. Environ. Contam. Toxicol.* 25:134–42.

Ho, M. W., Ryan, A., and Cummins, J. (2000). Hazards of transgenic plants containing the cauliflower mosaic virus promoter. *Microb. Ecol. Health. Dis.* 12(3):189–198.

Hodgson, J. (2000). Scientists avert new GMO crisis. *Nat. Biotechnol.* 18:13.

Hohlweg, U., and Doerfler, W. (2001). On the fate of plant or other foreign genes upon the uptake in food or after intramuscular injection in mice. *Mol. Genet. Genomics* 265:225–233.

Jennings, J. C., Kolwyck, D. C., Kays, S. B., Whetsell, A. J., Surber,

J. B., Cromwell, G. L., Lirette, R. P., and Glenn, K. C. (2003). Determining whether transgenic and endogenous plant DNA transgenic protein are detectable in muscle from swine fed Roundup Ready soybean meal. *J. Anim. Sci.* 81:1447– 1455.

Jennings, J. C., Albee, L. D., Kolwyck, D. C., Surber, J. B., Taylor, M. L., Hartnell, G. F., Lirette, R. P., and Glenn Monsanto, K. C. (2003b). Attempts to detect transgenic and endogenous plant DNA and transgenic protein in muscle from broilers fed YieldGard Corn Borer Corn. *Poult. Sci.* 82:371– 380.

Kuiper, H. A., Konig, A., Kleter, G. A., Hammes, W. P., Knudsen, I. (2004). Concluding remarks. Food Chem. *Toxicol.* 42:1195–1202.

Li, Y., Piao, J., Zhuo, Q., Chen, X., Mao, D., Yang, L., and Yang, X. (2004). *Study on the teratogenicity effects of genetically modified rice with Xa21 on rats* [in Chinese]. Wei Sheng Y an Jiu 33:710–2.

Liener, I. E. (1994). Implications of anti-nutritional components in soybean foods. *Crit. Rev. Food Sci. Nutr.* 34:31–67.

MacKenzie, S. A., Lamb, I., Schmidt, J., Deege, L., Morrisey, M. J., Harper, M., Layton, R. J., Prochaska, L. M., Sanders, C., Locke, M., Mattsson, J. L., Fuentes, A., and Delaney, B. (2007). Thirteen week feeding study with transgenic maize grain containing event DAS-Ø15Ø7-1 in Sprague–Dawley rats. *Food Chem. Toxicol.* 45:551–562.

Malatesta, M., Caporaloni, C., Gavaudan, S., Rocchi, M. B. L., Serafini, S.,

Tiberi, C., and Gazzanelli, G. (2002). Ultrastructural morphometrical and immunocytochemical analyses of hepatocyte nuclei from mice fed on genetically modified soybean. *Cell Struct. Funct.* 2:173-180.

Malatesta, M., Caporaloni, C., Rossi, L., Battistelli, S., Rocchi, M., and Tonucci, F. (2003). Ultrastructural analysis of pancreatic acinar cells from mice fed on genetically modified soybean. *J. Anat.* 201:409–415.

Malatesta, M., Tiberi, C., Baldelli, B., Battistelli, S., Manuali, E., and Biggiogera, M. (2005). Reversibility of hepatocyte nuclear modifications in mice fed on genetically modified soybean. *Eur. J. Histochem.* 49:237–42.

Margulis, C. (2006). The hazards of genetically engineered foods. *Environ. Health Perspect.* 114:A146–A147.

Martin, S. A. M., Vilhelmsson, O., M´edale, F., Watt, P., Kaushik, S., and Houlihan, D. F.(2003). Proteomic sensitivity to dietary manipulations in rainbow trout. *Biochim. Biophys. Acta* 1651:17–29.

Metcalfe, D. D., Astwood, J. D., Townsend, R., Sampson, H. A., Taylor, S. L., and Fuchs, R. L. (1996). Assessment of the allergenic potential of foods derived from genetically engineered crop plants. *Crit. Rev. Food Sci. Nutr.* 36:s165–s186.

Metcalfe, D. D. (2003). Introduction: What are the issues in addressing the allergenic potential of genetically modified foods? Environ. Health Perspect. 11:1110–1113.

Millstone, E., Brunner, E., and Mayer, S. (1999). Beyond "substantial equivalence." *Nature* 401:525–526.

Morris K. (1999). Bovine somatotropin—who's crying over spilt milk? Lancet 353:306.

Murray, S. R., Butler, R. C., Hardacre, A. K., and Timmerman-Vaughan. (2007). Use of quantitative real-time PCR to estimate maize endogenous DNA degradation after cooking and extrusion or in food products. *J. Agric. Food Chem.* 55:2231–9.

Niemann, H., and Rath, D. (2001). Transgenic pigs expressing plant genes. *Theriogenology.* 56:1291–1304.

Netherwood, T., Mart´in-Or´ue, S. M., O'Donnell, A. G., Gockling, S., Graham, J., Mathers, J. C., and Gilbert, H. J. (2004). Assessing the survival of transgenic plant DNA in the human gastrointestinal tract. *Nat. Biotechnol.* 22:204–209.

Nordlee, J. A., Taylor, S. L., Townsend, J. A., Thomas, L. A., and Bush, R. K. (1996). Identification of a Brazil nut allergen in transgenic soybeans. *N. Engl. J. Med.* 334:688–92.

Ostaszewska, T., Dabrowski, K., Palacios, M. E., Olejniczak, M., and Wieczorek, M. (2005). Growth morphological changes in the digestive tract of rainbow trout (*Oncorhynchus mykiss*) pacu (*Piaractus mesopotamicus*) due to casein replacement with soybean proteins. *Aquaculture* 245:273–286.

Padgette, S. R., Kolacz, K. H., Delannay, X., Re, D.B., La Vallee, B.J., Tinius, C. N., Rhodes, W. K., Otero, Y. I., Barry, G. F., Eichholtz, D., Peschke, V. M., Nida, D. L., Taylor, N. B., and Kishore, G. M. (1995). Development, identification and characterisation of a glyphosate-tolerant soybean line. *Crop Sci.* 35:1451–1461.

Padgette, S. R., Taylor, N. B., Nida, D. L., Bailey, M. R., MacDonald, J., Holden, L. R., and Fuchs, R. L. (1996). The composition of glyphosate-tolerant soybean seeds is equivalent to that of conventional soybeans. *J. Nutr.* 126:702– 716.

Palombo, J. D., DeMichele, S. J., Liu, J. W., Bistrian, B. R, and Huang, Y.S. (2000). Comparison of growth and fatty acid metabolism in rats fed diets containing equal levels of gamma-linolenic acid from high gamma-linolenic acid canola oil or borage oil. *Lipids* 35:975–81.

Paparini, A., and Romano-Spica, V. (2004). Public health issues related with the consumption of food obtained from genetically modified organisms. *Biotechnol Annu. Rev.* 10:85–122.

Paparini, A., and Romano-Spica, V. (2006). Gene transfer and cauliflower mosaic virus promoter 35S activity in mammalian cells. *J. Environ. Sci. Health* B 41:437–49.

Peng, D., Chen, S., Ruan, L., Li, L., Yu, Z., and Sun, M. (2007). Safety assessment of transgenic Bacillus thuringiensis with VIP insecticidal protein gene by feeding studies. *Food Chem. Toxicol.* Jan 11 [Epub ahead of print].

Phipps, R. H., and Beever, D. E. (2001). Detection of transgenic DNA in bovine milk: Preliminary results for cows receiving a TMR containing Yieldguard TM MON810. *Proc Int Anim Agr Food Sci Conf Indianapolis* (July 2001), p Abst. 476.

Poulsen, M., Kroghsbo, S., Schröder, M., Wilcks, A., Jacobsen, H., Miller, A., Frenzel, T., Danier, J., Rychlik, M., Shu, Q., Emami, K., Sudhakar, D., Gate-house, A., Engel, K.-H., and Knudsen, I. (2007). A 90-day safety study in Wistar rats fed genetically modified rice expressing snowdrop lectin Galanthus nivalis (GNA). *Food Chem. Toxicol.* 45:350–363.

Prescott, V. E., and Hogan, S. P. (2005). Genetically modified plants and food hypersensitivity diseases: Usage and implications of experimental models for risk assessment. *Pharmacol. Therap.* 111:374–383.

Prescott, V. E., Campbell, P. M., Mattes, J., Rothenberg, M. E., Foster, P. S., H. T. J. V. (2005). Transgenic expression of bean alpha-amylase inhibitor in peas results in altered structure immunogenicity. *J. Agric. Food Chem.* 53:9023–9030.

Pursel, V. G., Pinkert, C. A., Miller, K. F., Bolt, D. J., Campbell, R. G., Palmiter, R. D., Brinster, R. L., Hammer, R. E. (1989). Genetic engineering of livestock. *Science.* 244:1281–1288.

Pusztai, A., Bardocz, S., and Ewen, S. W. B. (2003). Genetically Modified Foods: Potential Human Health Effects. In: *Food Safety: Contaminants and Toxins* (ed) D'Mello JPF CAB International, Wallingford Oxon, UK, pp 347–372.

Rasmussen, R. S., and Morrissey, M. T. (2007). Biotechnology in aquaculture: transgenics and polyploidy. *Comprehensive Reviews in Food Science and Food Safety.* 6:2–16.

Rhee, G. S., Cho, D. H, Won, Y. H., Seok, J. H., Kim, S. S., Kwack, S. J., Lee, R. D., Chae, S. Y., Kim, J. W., Lee, B. M., Park, K. L., and

Choi, K. S. (2005). Multigeneration reproductive and developmental toxicity study of bar gene inserted into genetically modified potato on rats. *J. Toxicol. Environ. Health* 68:2263–76.

Richards, H. A., Chung-Ting Han, R. G., Hopkins, M. L., Failla, W. W., Ward, C. N., and Stewart Jr. (2003). Safety assessment of recombinant green fluorescent protein orally administered to weaned rats nutrient interactions and toxicity. *J. Nutr.* 133:1909–12.

Saeki, K., Matsumoto, K., Kinoshita, M., Suzuki, I., Tasaka, Y., Kano, K. et al. (2004). Functional expression of a Delta12 fatty acid desaturase gene from spinach in transgenic pigs. *Proc. Natl. Acad. Sci.* USA 101:6361–6366.

Sanden, M., Bruceb, I. J., Azizur Rahmanb, M., and Gro-Ingrunn Hemrea, M. (2004). The fate of transgenic sequences present in genetically modified plant products in fish feed, investigating the survival of GM soybean DNA fragments during feeding trials in Atlantic salmon, *Salmo salar* L. *Aquaculture* 237:391–405.

Schubbert, R., Renz, D., Schmitz, B., and Doerfler, W. (1997). Foreign (M13) DNA ingested by mice reaches peripheral leukocytes, spleen, liver via the intestinal wall mucosa can be covalently linked to mouse DNA. *Proc. Natl. Acad. Sci. USA* 94:961–966.

Scutt, C. P., Zubko, E., and Meyer, P. (2002). Techniques for the removal of marker genes from transgenic plants. *Biochimie* 84:1119–1126.

Seralini, G. E., Cellier, D., and de Venomois, J. S. (2007). New analysis of a rat feeding study with a genetically modified maize reveals signs of hepatorenal toxicity. *Arch. Environ. Contam. Toxicol.* Mar 13; [Epub ahead of print].

Singh, A. K., Mehta, A. K., Sridhara, S., Gaur, S. N., Singh, B. P., Sarma, P. U., and Arora, N. (2006). Allergenicity assessment of transgenic mustard (*Brassica juncea*) expressing bacterial codA gene. *Allergy.* 61:491–7.

Solomon, M. B., Pursel, V. G., Campbell, R. G., and Steele, N. C. (1997). Biotechnology for porcine products and its effect on meat products. *Food Chem.* 59:499–504

Sayanova, O., Smith, M. A., Lapinskas, P., Stobart, A. K., Dobson, G., and Christie, W. W. (1997). Expression of a borage desaturase cDNA containing an N-terminal cytochrome b5 domain results in the accumulation of high levels of delta6-desaturated fatty acids in transgenic tobacco. *Proc. Natl. Acad. Sci. USA* 94:4211–6.

Strieber W. (2002). *Unknown country. Even Pigs Can't Survive on GM Corn.* www. unknowncountry.com/news/?id=1689.

Taylor, S. L., and Hefle, S. L. (2002). Genetically engineered foods: implications for food allergy. *Curr. Opin. Allergy Clin. Immunol.* 2:249–52.

Tepfer, M., Gaubert, S., Leroux-Coyau, M., Prince, S., and Houdebine, L. M. (2004). Transient expression in mammalian cells of transgenes transcribed from the Cauliflower mosaic virus 35S promoter. *Environ. Biosafety Res.* 3:91–7.

Teshima, R., Watanabe, T., Olunuki, H., Isuzugawa, K., Akiyama, H., Onodera, H., Imai, T., Toyoda, M., and Sawada, J.-I. (2002). Effect of subchronic feeding of genetically modified corn (CBH351) on immune system in BN rats and B10A mice. *Shokuhin Eiseigaku Zasshi.* 43:273–9.

Tryphonas, H., Arvanitakis G., Vavasour E., and Bondy G. (2003). Animal models to detect allergenicity to foods and genetically modified products: Workshop summary. *Environ. Health Perspect.* 11:221–222.

Van Neerven, R. J. J., Wikborg, T., Lund, G., Jacobsen, B., Brinch-Nielsen, A., and Arnved, J. (1999). Blocking antibodies induced by specific allergy vaccination prevent the activation of CD4+ T cells by inhibiting serum-IgE-facilitated allergen presentation. *J. Immunol.* 163:2944– 52.

Varzakas, T. H., Arvanitoyannis, I. S., and Baltas H. The politics and science behind GMO acceptance. *Crit. Rev.Food Sci. Nutr.* 47:335–361.

Vazquez-Padron, R. I., Moreno-Fierros, L., Neri-Baz´an, L., A. de la Riva, G., and L´opez-Revilla, R. (1999). Intragastric and intraperitoneal administration of Cry1Ac protoxin from Bacillus thuringiensis induces systemic mucosal antibody responses in mice. *Life Sci.* 64:1897–1912.

Vazquez-Padron, R.I., Gonz´ales-Cabrera, J., Garc´ia-Tovar, C., Neri-Bazan, L.,Lop´ez-Revilla, R., and Hern´andez, M. (2000). Cry1Ac protoxin from Bacillus thuringiensis sp. Kurstaki HD73 binds to surface proteins in the mouse small intestine. *Biochem. Biophys. Res. Commun.* 271:54–58.

Weil, J. H. (2005). Are genetically modified plants useful and safe? *IUBMB Life* 57:311–314.

Zhuo, Q., Chen, X., Piao, J., and Gu, L. (2004). [Study on food safety of genetically modified rice which expressed cowpea trypsin inhibitor by 90 day feeding test on rats]. *Wei Sheng Yan Jiu* 33:176–9.

Supportive References

Organically certified foods of both animal and plant origin contain more essential nutrients, notably antioxidants, than conventionally grown produce, and of course cause less environmental harms and are pesticide and GE/GM free. For documentation, see Cooper J, Leifert C, and Niggily U, (eds) *Handbook of Food Quality and Safety*, Cambridge, UK, Woodhead Publ. Inc. 2007.

Benachour, N. H. et al., Time- and Dose-Dependent Effects of Roundup on Human Embryonic and Placental Cells, *Archives of Environmental Contamination and Toxicology*, online: 4 May 2007.

Benbrook, C. "Genetically Engineered Crops and Pesticide Use in the United States: The First Nine Years"; *BioTech InfoNet*, Technical Paper Number 7, October 2004.

Chowdhury, E. H., et al., Detection of corn intrinsic and recombinant DNA fragments Cry1Ab protein in the gastrointestinal contents of pigs fed genetically modified corn Bt11. *J. Anim. Sci.* 81:2546–2551.2003.

Doerfler, W., and Schubbert R. Uptake of foreign DNA from the environment: the gastro-intestinal tract the placenta as portals of entry. *Wien Klin. Wochenschr* 110:40–44. 1998.

Domingo, José L. 'Toxicity Studies of Genetically Modified Plants: A Review of the Published Literature', *Critical Reviews in Food Science and Nutrition*, 47:8, 721 – 733, 2007.

Dona, A., and I.S. Arvanitoyannis, Health Risks of Genetically Modified Foods. *Critical Reviews in Food Science and Nutrition.* 49: 164-175, 2009.

Ermakova, I. *Genetically modified soy affects posterity: Results of Russian scientists' studies.* Available online at: http://www.geneticsafety.org/info.php?txt-id=19&nid=776. 2005.

Ermakova, I., "Genetically modified soy leads to the decrease of weight and high mortality of rat pups of the first generation. Preliminary studies," *Ecosinform* 1 (2006): 4–9. pp.4-9 (in Russian).

Ewen, S. W. B., and Pusztai, A. Effect of diets containing genetically modified potatoes expressing Galanthus nivalis lectin on rat small intestine. *Lancet* 354:1353–1354.1999.

Fares, N. H., and El-Sayed, A. K. Fine structural changes in the ileum of mice fed on delta-endotoxin-treated potatoes and transgenic potatoes. *Natural Toxins* 6:219–233 1998.

Finamore, A., et al, Intestinal and peripheral immune response to MON810 maize ingestion in weaning and old mice. *J Agric Food*

Chem, http://pubs.ac.org, 16 November 2008.

Fox, M.W., E. Hodgkins and M. Smart, *Not Fit For A Dog: The Truth About Manufactured Dog and Cat Food*. Sanger, CA., Quill Driver Books, 2009.

Fox, M.W., *Killer Foods: What Scientists Do To Make Better is not Always Best*. Gulford, CT, The Lyons Press, 2004.

Germolec, D. R., Kimber, I., Goldman, L., and Selgrade. Key issues for the assessment of the allergenic potential of genetically modified foods: Breakout group reports. *Environ. Health Perspect* 11:1131–1139. 2003.

Ho, M. W., Ryan, A., and Cummins, J. Hazards of transgenic plants containing the cauliflower mosaic virus promoter. *Microb. Ecol. Health. Dis.* 12(3):189–198. 2000.

Kilic, A. and M. T. Akay. A three generation study with genetically modified Bt corn in rats: Biochemical and histopathological investigation. *Food Chem. Toxicol.* 46(3): 1164-1170.2008.

Leeson, S., "The Effect of Glufosinate Resistant Corn on Growth of Male Broiler Chickens," *Department of Animal and Poultry Sciences, University of Guelph, Report No. A56379,* July 12, 1996.

Liener, I. E. Implications of anti-nutritional components in soybean foods. *Crit. Rev. Food Sci. Nutr.* 34:31–67. 1994.

Malatesta, M. et al., Fine Structural Analyses of Pancreatic Acinar Cell Nuclei from Mice Fed on GM Soybean, *Eur J Histochem* 47: 385–388.2003.

Malatesta, M., et al, Reversibility of Hepatocyte Nuclear Modifications in Mice Fed on Genetically Modified Soybean, *Eur J Histochem*, 49: 237-242 2005.

Malatesta, M., et al, Hepatoma tissue culture (HTC) cells as a model for investigating the effects of low concentrations of herbicide on cell structure and function (Roundup residues interfere with multiple metabolic pathways?). *Toxicol In Vitro.* 2008 Sep 18;: 18835430 (P,S,G,E,B,D)

Oliveri, et al., "Temporary Depression of Transcription in Mouse Pre-implantion Embryos from Mice Fed on Genetically Modified Soybean," *48th Symposium of the Society for Histochemistry*, Lake Maggiore (Italy), September 7–10, 2006.

Paparini, A., and Romano-Spica, V. Gene transfer and cauliflower mosaic virus promoter 35S activity in mammalian cells. J. Environ. *Sci. Health B* 41:437–49. 2006.

Pusztai, A., Bardocz, S., and Ewen, S. W. B. Genetically Modified Foods: Potential Human Health Effects. In: *Food Safety: Contaminants and*

Toxins (ed) D'Mello JPF CAB International, Wallingford Oxon, UK, pp 347–372 2003.

Schubbert, R., Renz, D., Schmitz, B., and Doerfler, W. Foreign (M13) DNA ingested by mice reaches peripheral leukocytes, spleen, liver via the intestinal wall mucosa can be covalently linked to mouse DNA. *Proc. Natl. Acad. Sci. USA* 94:961–966. 1997.

Seralini, G. E., Cellier, D., and de Venomois, J. S. New analysis of a rat feeding study with genetically modified maize reveals signs of hepatorenal toxicity. *Arch. Environ. Contam. Toxicol.* Mar 13; [Epub ahead of print]. 2007.

Smith J. M, *Genetic Roulette: The Documented Health Risks of Genetically Engineered Foods*, and visit his website www.seedsofdeception.com.

Tepfer, M., Gaubert, S., Leroux-Coyau, M., Prince, S., and Houdebine, L. M. Transient expression in mammalian cells of transgenes transcribed from the Cauliflower mosaic virus 35S promoter. *Environ. Biosafety Res.* 3:91–7. 2004.

Traavik, T., and Jack Heinemann, J., Genetic Engineering and Omitted Health Research: Still No Answers to Ageing Questions, *TWN Biotechnology & Biosafety Series 7*, 2007.

Tudisco, R., et al, Genetically Modified Soya Bean in Rabbit Feeding: Detection of DNA Fragments and Evaluation of Metabolic Effects by Enzymatic Analysis, *Animal Science* 82: 193–199, 2006.

Vecchio, L., et al, "Ultrastructural Analysis of Testes from Mice Fed on Genetically Modified Soybean," *European Journal of Histochemistry* 48, no. 4 (Oct–Dec 2004):449–454.

Velimirov, A, Binter C and Zentek J. Biological effects of transgenic maize NK603xMON810 fed in long term reproduction studies in mice. *Report, Forschungsberichte der Sektion IV, Band 3. Institut für Ernährung, and Forschungsinstitut für biologischen Landbau,* Vienna, Austria, November 2008.http://www.bmgfj.gv.at/cms/site/attachments/3/2/9/CH0810/

Wilson, A.K, J.R. Latham, and R.A. Steinbrecher, 'Transformation-induced mutations in transgenic plants: Analysis and biosafety implications. *Biotechnology and Genetic Engineering Reviews*, 23, p 209-226, 2006.

Additional Notes & References

Prepared by Dr. Brian John, GM Free Cymru. Wales, UK.

Ewen SWB, Pusztai A (1999) Effect of diets containing genetically modified potatoes expressing Galanthus nivalis lectin on rat small intestine. *Lancet* 354:1353-1354.

The Flavr-Savr tomato was withdrawn in 1996, amid claims that it was a commercial failure. So was another variety called Endless Summer. But trials of the Flavr-Savr tomato showed there were health concerns which contributed to the "commercial" decision. http://www.soilassociation.org/web/sa/saweb.nsf/0/80256cad0046ee0c80 256d1f005b0ce5?OpenDocument

The StarLink maize fiasco occurred in 2000 and is well documented. See also: http://www.i-sis.org.uk/biotechdebacle_updated.php

A new GM soya was developed, containing genes from Brazil nuts (1996). A novel protein was accidentally created which had the potential to affect people with nut allergies—so the GM soya was withdrawn: http://www.health24.com/dietnfood/Food_causing_disease/15-737-740,32410.asp

As a consequence of the L-tryptophan scandal (1989) there were c 100 deaths (Jeffrey Smith). Seethese:>http://www.responsibletechnology.org/utility/showArticle/?objectID=283&find=L%2Dtryptophan www.seedsofdeception.com/Public/L-tryptophan/index.cfm

Fares NH, El-Sayed AK. 1998. Fine structural changes in the ileum of mice fed on delta-endotoxin-treated potatoes and transgenic potatoes. *Nat Toxins*. 6:219-33.

The rBGH bovine growth hormone (BST) has been promoted globally by Monsanto in the full knowledge of science showing damage to both cattle and those who consume the milk of cows treated with rBGH. http://www.responsibletechnology.org/utility/showArticle/? ObjectID=193&find=BST

The deaths of cattle in Hesse, Germany, have been linked with Bt176 maize, but there appear to have been determined efforts to "lose" key scientific information and to attribute the cattle deaths to mismanagement and other factors. http://www.i-sis.org.uk/CAGMMAD.php

Broiler chickens fed on Chardon LL—the mortality rate was twice as high as that of the control group (NB the infamous case of Prof Alan Gray of ACRE and the failure of that Committee to examine evidence placed before it. ...) http://www.i-sis.org.uk/appeal.php

Rats fed on Chardon LL—weight gain was much reduced http://www.i-sis.org.uk/appeal.php
The work of the Norwegian scientist Terje Traavik and his colleagues is on-going and has still to be published. But see: "Filipino islanders blame GM crop for mystery sickness. Monsanto denies scientist's claim that maize may have caused 100 villagers to fall ill"—John Aglionby in Kalyong, southern Philippines, *The Guardian*, Wednesday 3 March 3, 2004. http://www.guardian.co.uk/gmdebate/Story/0,2763,1160789,00.html
Allergic reactions and livestock deaths 2005 attributable to Bt cotton In India (Madhya Pradesh):http://news.webindia123.com/news/showdetails.asp?id=170692&cat=Health
The Newcastle feeding study (published 2003) involved a small portion of GM soya fed to just seven ileostomy patients: http://www.foodstandards.gov.uk/news/newsarchive/statement http://www.gmwatch.org/archive2.asp?arcid=990
Re the Monsanto rat feeding study on MON863 maize, which the company was desperate to keep out of the public domain (2004): http://www.seedsofdeception.com/utility/showArticle/?objectID=221 Genetically Modified Corn Study Reveals Health Damage and Cover-up, by Jeffrey M. Smith http://news.independent.co.uk/world/science_technology/story.jsp?story=640430 http://www.efsa.eu.int/science/gmo/gmo_opinions/381_en.html http://www.gmwatch.org/archive2.asp?arcid=5270
The regulatory system for GM crops and foodstuffs is a disgrace, and needs to be scrapped and replaced. The GM authorizations process in both Europe and the USA is underpinned by the scientifically nonsensical concept of "substantial equivalence," by which a cow with BSE would be considered to be "substantially equivalent" to one without. Further, the authorities depend almost exclusively upon the "science" submitted by the biotechnology corporations with their applications, which is almost always partial and selective. In other words, it is corrupt. Again, the regulatory process is designed - quite specifically - to facilitate authorizations rather than to protect the consumer. The regulatory bodies themselves are packed with placements from the GM industry—people whose very careers depend upon a continuation of the GM enterprise. The precautionary principle, which is supposed to underpin the regulatory process, has now been effectively replaced by the "anti-precautionary principle," by

which GMs are assumed to be harmless unless opponents can prove otherwise, on a variety-specific basis. But independent scientists cannot undertake effective research because the genetic constructs of new GM varieties are closely guarded secrets, and because governments will not fund their studies. And finally, in Europe at least, the Commission is more concerned about politics than science, and is determined to issue GM authorizations, come hell or high water, just to show the Americans and the WTO that there is no GM moratorium in place.

It should also be added that recent studies have shown that the pollen from various types of Bt corn/maize will kill caterpillars and other insects when the wind-blown pollen settles on the leaves of other plants; and that both Bt corn and Bt cotton crop residues contaminate the soil with Bt toxin.

Jeffrey M. Smith, who publishes "Spilling The Beans," a monthly column available at www.responsibletechnology.org. writes that: It turns out that the damage done to DNA due to the process of creating a genetically modified organism is far more extensive than previously thought.[1] GM crops routinely create unintended proteins, alter existing protein levels or even change the components and shape of the protein that is created by the inserted gene. The concerns of Kirk Azevedo, former Monsanto employee and whistle blower (who left the company after his concerns about their GM crop varieties producing harmful misfolded proteins, which he felt were in some ways analogous to the misfolded prions responsible for Mad Cow disease, fell on deaf ears), have been echoed by other scientists as one of many possible dangers that are not being evaluated by the biotech industry's superficial safety assessments.

GM cotton has provided ample reports of unpredicted side-effects. In April 2006, more than 70 Indian shepherds reported that 25% of their herds died within 5-7 days of continuous grazing on Bt cotton plants. [2] Hundreds of Indian agricultural laborers reported allergic reactions from Bt cotton. Some cotton harvesters have been hospitalized and many laborers in cotton gin factories take antihistamines each day before work. [3]

The cotton's agronomic performance is also erratic. When Monsanto's GM cotton varieties were first introduced in the US, tens of thousands of acres suffered deformed roots and other unexpected problems. Monsanto paid out millions in settlements.[4] When Bt cotton was tested in Indonesia, widespread pest infestation and drought damage forced withdrawal of the crop, despite the fact that Monsanto had been bribing at least 140 individuals for years, trying to gain approval.[5] In India, inconsistent performance has resulted in more than $80 million dollars in losses in each of two states.[6] Thousands of indebted Bt cotton farmers have committed suicide. In Vidarbha, in north east Maharashtra, from June through August 2006, farmers committed suicide at a rate of about one every eight hours.[7] (The list of adverse reactions reported from other GM crops, in lab animals, livestock and humans, is considerably longer.)

Kirk's concern about GM crop test plots also continues to remain valid. The industry has been consistently inept at controlling the spread of unapproved varieties. On August 18, 2006, for example, the USDA announced that unapproved GM long grain rice, which was last field tested by Bayer CropScience in 2001, had contaminated the US rice crop[8] (probably for the past 5 years). Japan responded by suspending long grain rice imports and the EU will now only accept shipments that are tested and certified GM-free. Similarly, in March 2005, the US government admitted that an unapproved corn variety had escaped from Syngenta's field trials four years earlier and had contaminated US corn.[9] By year's end, Japan had rejected at least 14 shipments containing the illegal corn. Other field trialed crops have been mixed with commercial varieties, consumed by farmers, stolen, even given away by government agencies and universities who had accidentally mixed seed varieties.

Some contamination from field trials may last for centuries. That may be the fate of a variety of unapproved Roundup Ready grass which, according to reports made public in August 2006, had escaped into the wild from an Oregon test plot years earlier. Pollen had crossed with other varieties and wind had dispersed seeds. Scientists believe that the variety will cross pollinate with other grass varieties and may contaminate the commercial grass seed supply—70 percent of which is grown in Oregon.

Even GM crops with known poisons are being grown outdoors without adequate safeguards for health and the environment. A corn engineered to produce pharmaceutical medicines, for example, contaminated corn and soybean fields in Iowa and Nebraska in 2002.[10] On August 10, 2006, a federal judge ruled that the drug-producing GM crops grown in Hawaii violated both the Endangered Species Act and the National Environmental Policy Act.[11]

A December 29, 2005 report by the USDA office of Inspector General, blasted the agriculture department for its abysmal oversight of GM field trials, particularly for the high risk drug producing crops. [12] And a January 2004 report by the National Research Council also called upon the government to strengthen its oversight, but acknowledged that there is no way to guarantee that field trialed crops will not pollute the environment.[13]

With the US government failing to prevent GM contamination, and with state governments and agriculture commissioners unwilling to challenge the dictates of the biotech industry, some California counties decided to enact regulations of their own. California's diverse agriculture is particularly vulnerable and thousands of field trials on not-yet-approved GM crops have already taken place there. If contamination were discovered, it could easily devastate an industry.

Four counties have enacted moratoria or bans on the planting of GM crops, including both approved and unapproved varieties. This follows the actions of more than 4500 jurisdictions in Europe and dozens of nations, states and regions on all continents, which have sought to restrict planting of GM crops to protect their health, environment and agriculture.

Jeffrey Smith's book, *Genetic Roulette*, documents more than 60 health risks of GM foods in easy-to-read two-page spreads, and demonstrates how current safety assessments are not competent to protect consumers from the dangers. His previous book, Seeds of Deception (www.seedsofdeception.com), is the world's bestselling book on the subject.

Spilling the Beans is a monthly column available at www. responsibletechnology.org

Notes for Previous References from Dr. John

[1] JR Latham et al., "The Mutational Consequences of Plant Transformation," *The Journal of Biomedicine and Biotechnology*, Vol. 2006 Article ID 25376 Pages 1-7, DOI 10.1155/JBB/2006/25376; for a more in-depth discussion, see also Allison Wilson et al., "Genome Scrambling -Myth or Reality? Transformation-Induced Mutations in Transgenic Crop Plants, Technical Report - October 2004, www. econexus.info.

[2] Mortality in Sheep Flocks after Grazing on Bt Cotton Fields – Warangal District, Andhra Pradesh. *Report of the Preliminary Assessment* April 2006,

http://www.gmwatch.org/archive2.asp?arcid=6494

[3] Ashish Gupta, et. al., Impact of Bt Cotton on Farmers' Health (in Barwani and Dhar District of Madhya Pradesh), *Investigation Report*, Oct - Dec 2005

[4] See for example, Monsanto Cited In Crop Losses *New York Times*, June 16, 1998,http://query.nytimes.com/gst/fullpage.html?res=9A04E ED6153DF935A25755C0A96E958260; and Greenpeace http:// archive.greenpeace.org/geneng/reports/gmo/intrgmo5.htm

[5] Antje Lorch, Monsanto Bribes in Indonesia, Monsanto Fined For Bribing Indonesian Officials to Avoid Environmental Studies for Bt Cotton, ifrik 1sep2005, http://www.mindfully.org/GE/2005/ Monsanto-Bribes-Indonesia1sep05.htm

[6] Bt Cotton - No Respite for Andhra Pradesh Farmers More than 400 crores' worth losses for Bt Cotton farmers in *Kharif 2005 Centre for Sustainable Agriculture: Press Release*, March 29, 2006 http://www. gmwatch.org/archive2.asp?arcid=6393; see also November 14, 2005 article in www.NewKerala.com regarding Madhya Pradesh.

[7] Jaideep Hardikar, One suicide every 8 hours, *Daily News & Analysis* (India), August 26, 2006 http://www.dnaindia.com/report. asp?NewsID=1049554

[8] Rick Weiss, U.S. Rice Supply Contaminated, Genetically Altered Variety Is Found in Long-Grain Rice, *Washington Post*, August 19, 2006.

[9] Jeffrey Smith, US Government and Biotech Firm Deceive Public on GM Corn Mix-up, Spilling the Beans, April 2005.

[10] See for example, Christopher Doering, ProdiGene to spend millions on bio-corn tainting, *Reuters News Service*, USA: December 9, 2002

[11] See www.centerforfoodsafety.org

[12] Office of Inspector General, USDA, *Audit Report Animal and Plant Health Inspection Service Controls Over Issuance of Genetically Engineered Organism Release Permits*, December 2005 http://www.thecampaign. org/USDA_IG_1205.pdf

[13] Justin Gillis, Genetically Modified Organisms Not Easily Contained; National Research Council Panel Urges More Work to Protect Against Contamination of Food Supply, *Washington Post*, Jan 21, 2004.

Research continues to support the urgent need to adopt organic farming methods, as per the findings of L. Ozturk et al. (*New Phytologist*, 2007) that the iron deficiency increasingly observed in major crops is associated with the application of the herbicide glyphosate, which interferes with plants' uptake of iron from the soil. Manganese uptake is also impaired.

Humans are Guinea Pigs for the "Second Generation" of Genetically-Modified(GM) Crops

In an October 15th, 2009 press release, CRIIGEN (Committee for Independent Research and Information on Genetic Engineering at www. criigen.org) denounced the scandalous approval of a new GM maize variety in Europe named 59122xNK603. Governments and industry have promised a "second generation" of GM crops in the service of humanity. For example crops tolerant to harsh environmental conditions such as drought, flooding and salinity caused by climate change to help combat world hunger. However, the reality is quite different. Instead these supposedly new second generation crops are simply more sophisticated versions of the old ones producing several insecticides and absorbing several herbicides. The 59122xNK603 maize is a GM crop powerhouse of four pesticides (two insecticides and two herbicides) with cumulative and compounding health and environmental risks as is inherently the case with the new Canadian GM maize SmartStax, which ultimately can contain up to eight different pesticides!

Furthermore, to avoid calls for transparency and availability of results obtained from previous investigations addressing the health consequences of eating GM crops and foods, governments, agricultural biotech seed and pesticide firms have decided to dispense altogether with animal feeding studies ... instead they now prefer to test GM foods directly on the public!

This new generation of GM 'SmartStax' maize (corn), containing eight novel traits, developed jointly by Monsanto and Dow Agrosciences, was approved in the US by the Food and Drug Administration in the absence of new safety assessments according to the AgBiotech Reporter (Aug 10th, 2009, p11) (www.foodregulation.com).

Adding support to the American Academy of Environmental medicine position paper calling for an immediate moratorium on GM foods that pose a "serious health risk" (stating that "Multiple animal studies have shown that GM foods cause damage to various organ systems of the body"), the Union of Concerned Scientists released a report in the fall of 2009 entitled Failure to Yield, that documented the superior yields of conventional crops. (www.ucsusa.org/food_and_agriculture).

CHAPTER 12

American Association of Veterinarians for Animal Rights, *Guide to Congenital and Hereditary Disorders in Dogs*. P.O. Box 208, Davis, CA 95617-0208.

Bauer, John E. Responses of Dogs to Omega-3 Fatty Acids. *J. Amer. Vet. Med. Assoc.*, 231:1657-1661, 2007.

Campbell, T.C, *The China Study*: The most comprehensive study of nutrition conducted, and the startling implication for diet, weight-loss and long-term health. Dallas TX Bell Bella Books, 2005.

Dye, J.A. et al, Elevated PBDE levels in pet cats: sentinels for humans? *Environmental Science & Technology*, 41: 6350-6356, 2007.

Fox, M.W, Veterinary Bioethics, pp 673-678 in *Complementary and Alternative Medicine*, A.M. Schoen and S.G. Wynn, eds, Mosby, St Lois, MO 1997.

Heinemann, K.M. and J.E. Bauer, Docosahexaenoic acid and neurologic development in animals. *J. Amer. Vet. Med. Assoc.*, 228:700-705, 2006.

McMichael, M.A., Oxidative stress, antioxidants, and assessment of oxidative stress in dogs and cats. *J. Amer. Vet. Med. Assoc.*, 231: 734-720, 2007.

News/Companion Animals, Top 10 reasons pets visit veterinarians, *Journal of the American Veterinary Medical Assoc*, Sept 1, vol.229, p 651, 2006.

News and Reports. Rats reveal risks of 'junk food' during pregnancy. *The Veterinary Record*, Aug 18, p 215, 2007.

Platinga, E.A, et al, Retrospective study of the survival of cats with acquired chronic renal insufficiency offered different commercial diets. *The Veterinary Record*, Vol. 157: p455-6, 2005.

Roudebush, P. et al Nutritional management of brain aging dogs. *J. Amer. vet. Med. Assoc.*227:722-728, 2006.

Steinfeld, H, P. Gerber P, Wassenaer T, Castel V, Rosales M, and de Haan C. *Livestock's Long Shadow: Environmental Losses and Options*. United Nation's Food and Agriculture Organization, Washington, DC, 2006.

Caution is called for especially with cats, when using household cleaners and other chemical products. See Alexandra Gorman, *Household Hazards: Potential Hazards of Home Cleaning Products*. A report by the Women's Voice for the Earth, 2007

Note: a common flame retardant, polybrominated diphenyl ethers (PBDEs), used in carpet padding, fabrics and mattresses, and found to be at high levels in fish-flavored canned cat foods, has been

recently linked by the US Environmental Protection Agency, with hyperthyroidism in cats. PBDEs are endocrine disruptors like the PCBs and dioxins, high levels of all these being common in farmed salmon.(www.epa.gov/oppt/pbde).
For additional reading and documentation of manufactured pet food concerns, see *Not Fit for a Dog: The Truth About Manufactured Dog and Cat Food* by Drs. Michael W. Fox, Elizabeth Hodgkins, and Marion E. Smart, Quill Driver Books, Sanger, CA. 2008.

CHAPTER 13

For more details on this modern food crisis and its adverse effects on companion animals, see *Not Fit For A Dog: The Truth About Manufactured Dog And Cat Food* by veterinarians Drs. M.W. Fox, E. Hodgkins, and M. E. Smart, published in 2008 by Quill Driver Books, Sanger, CA.
For further assurance and information, contact a holistic veterinarian in your area. A searchable list can be found at http://www.ahvma.org
Veterinarians wishing to learn more are encouraged to become members of the American Holistic Veterinary Medical Association at http://www.ahvma.org.)
Cooper J, Leifert C, and Niggily U, (eds). *Handbook of Organic Food Safety and Quality*, Cambridge, UK, Woodhead Publications 2007.

Some additional supportive citations

Domingo, J.L, Toxicity Studies of Genetically Modified Plants: A Review of Published Literature. *Critical Reviews in Food Science and Nutrition* 47:721-733, 2007.
Dona, A., and I.S. Arvanitoyannis, Health Risks of Genetically Modified Foods. *Critical reviews in Food Science and Nutrition*. 49: 164-175, 2008
Gallou-Kabani, C. and C. Junien, Nutritional Epigenomics of Metabolic Syndrome, New Perspective Against the Epidemic, *Diabetes* 54(2005): 1899–1906; see also J. E. Cropley, et al.,
Germ-line epigenetic modification of the murine Avy allele by nutritional supplementation, *Proc Natl Acad Sci U S A*.103, no. 46 (Nov 14, 2006):17308–17312.
German, A. J., and L.E. Morgan, How often do veterinarians assess bodyweight and body condition in dogs? *The Veterinary Record*. Oct 25, p 503- 506, 2008
Ludwig, D.S., and Pollack, D.S., Obesity and the Economy: from Crisis to

Opportunity. *JAMA*, 301: 533-535, 2009.

News and Reports: Rats reveal risks of 'junk food' during pregnancy. *The Veterinary Record*, Aug 18, p 215, 2007.

Robinson J. *Pasture Perfect: The Far-Reaching Benefits of Choosing Meat, Eggs, and Dairy Products from Grass-Fed Animals*. Vashon, WA, Vashon Island Press, 2004.

Smith J. M. *Genetic Roulette: The Documented Health Risks of Genetically Engineered Foods*, and visit his website www.seedsofdeception.com.

Sullivan K. *The Lectin Report*. 7/29/08 www.krispin.com/lectin.html

Symes, John B., DVM. *Food Intolerance in people and Pets*. www.dogtorj.net

Wilson, A.K, J.R. Latham and R.A. Steinbrecher, 'Transformation-induced mutations in transgenic plants: Analysis and biosafety implications. *Biotechnology and Genetic Engineering Reviews*, 23, p 209-226, 2006.

Selected References

Alexander, A. N., M. K. Huelsmeyer, A. Mitzey, R. R. Dubielzig, I. D. Kurzman, E. G. Macewen, and D. M. Vail. 2006. Development of an allogenic whole-cell tumor vaccine expressing xenogeneic gp100 and its implementation in a phase II clinical trial in canine patients with malignant melanoma. *Cancer Immunol. Immunother*. 55:433-442

American Veterinary Medical Association letter, re Center for Veterinary Biologics Notice Draft No. 327: Studies to Support Label Claims of Duration of Immunity dated October 27 2008: http://www.avma.org/advocacy/federal/regulatory/practice_issues/vaccines/duration_of_immunity_ltr.pdf

Azad, N., and Y. Rojanasakul. 2006. Vaccine delivery—current trends and future. *Curr. Drug Deliv*. 3:137-146.

Beck, M.A. 2000. Nutritionally induced oxidative stress: effect on viral disease. *Amer. J. Clinical Nutrition* 71: 1676S-1679s.

Bergman, P.J., McKnight, J., Novosad, A., Charney, S., Farrelly, J., Craft, D., Wulderk, M., Jeffers, Y., Sadelain, M., Hohenhaus, A.E., Segal, N., Gregor, P., Engelhorn, M., Riviere, I., Houghton, A.N., and Wolchok, J.D.. Long-term survival of dogs with advanced malignant melanoma after DNA vaccination with xenogeneic human tyrosinase: a phase I trial. *Clin Cancer Res*. 2003, 9(4), 1284-90.

Chan, V. Use of genetically modified viruses and genetically engineered virus-vector vaccines; Environmental effects. *J. Toxicology and Environmental Health Part A*. 69: 1 2006, pp. 1971-1977(7).

Classen, J.B. et al.1999 Association between type 1 diabetes and Hib vaccine *BMJ* 319:1133

Crawford, C. 2002. The Current Status of Canine Vaccinations: Are We Vaccinating Dogs with Too Many vaccines Too Often? *Dog Owners and Breeders Symposium*, University of Florida College of Veterinary Medicine.

Day, M.J., Horzinek, M.C., Schultz, R.D. Guidelines for the Vaccination of Dogs and Cats, compiled by the Vaccination Guidelines Group (VGG) of the World Small Animal Veterinary Association (WSAVA). *Journal of Small Animal Practice*. 2007. 48 (9), 528-541: http://www.wsava.org/PDF/Misc/VGG_09_2007.pdf

Delves, P.J., T. Lund, and I. M. Roitt. 2002. Antifertility vaccines. *Trends Immunol.* 23:213-219.

de Vries, J., Meier, P., and Wackernagel, W. 2004. Microbial horizontal gene transfer and the DNA release from transgenic crop plants. *Plant and Soil*, 266: 91-104.

Dodds, W.J. 2001. Vaccination protocols for dogs predisposed to vaccine reactions. *J Am Animal Hosp Assoc* 38: 1-4.

Duval, D. and U. Giger. 1996. Vaccine-Associated Immune-Mediated Hemolytic Anemia in the Dog, *Journal of Veterinary Internal Medicine* 10:290-295.

England, J. 2008. New Vaccine Technologies: Destined for Cattle Vaccines, *CVC Proceedings*. August 1st.

Fehiner-Gardiner, C., et al 2008. ERA vaccine-derived cases of rabies in wildlife and domestic animals in Ontario, Canada, 1989-2004. *J. Wildlife Diseases*, 44: 71-85.

Ford, R.B. 2001. Vaccines and Vaccination: The Strategic Issues. In: *North American Veterinary Clinics*. Ford, R.B., ed. 31: 439-453.

Frick, O.L., and D. L. Brooks. . 1983. Immunoglobilin E antibodies in pollen-augmented in dogs by virus vaccines. *Am. J. Vet Res.* 44: 440-445.

Friedrich, F. et al 1996. Temporal association between the isolation of Sabin-related poliovirus vaccine strains and the Guillan-Barre syndrome *Rev Inst Med Trop.* Sao Paulo, Jan-Feb; 38(1):55-8.

Hardham, J., M. Reed, J. Wong, K. King, B. Laurinat, C. Sfintescu, and R. T. Evans. 2005. Evaluation of a monovalent companion animal periodontal disease vaccine in an experimental mouse periodontitis model. *Vaccine* 23:3148-3156.

Hogenesch, H., and L.T. Glickmman. 1997. Effects of Vaccination on the Endocrine and Immune Systems of Dogs, Phase II," Purdue University, at http://www.homestead.com/vonhapsburg/

haywardstudyonvaccines.html. www.vet.purdue.edu/epi/gdhstudy.
htm.

Hogenesch, H., J. Azcona-Olivera, and C .Scott-Moncrieff, et al. 1999.
Vaccine-induced autoimmunity in the dog. *Adv Vet Med.* 41: 733-747.

Isaguliants, M.G., Iakimtchouk, K., Petrakova, N.V., Yermalovich, M.A.,
Zuber, A.K., Kashuba, V.I., Belikov, S.V., Andersson, S., Kochetkov,
S.N., Klinman. D.M., and Wahren, B. Gene immunization may
induce secondary antibodies reacting with DNA. *Vaccine* 2004, 22(11-
12),1576-85.

Kirpensteinjn, J. Feline injection site-associated sarcoma: Is it a reason to
critically evaluate our vaccination policies? *Vet Microbiol.* 2006, 117:
59-65.

Kowalczyk, D. and Ertl. H. Immune response to DNA vaccines. *CMLS
Cell. Mol. Life Sci.* 1999, 55, 751-70.

Kuiken, T., G. Rimmelzwaan, D. van Riel, G. van Amerongen, M. Baars,
R. Fouchier, and A. Osterhaus. 2004. Avian H5N1 influenza in cats.
Science 306:241.

Lappin, M.R., Basaraba RJ, Jensen WA. Interstitial nephritis in cats
inoculated with Crandell Rees feline kidney cell lysates. *J. Feline Med.
Surg.* 2006;8:353-356.

Lappin, M.R.,, Sebring RW, Porter M, Radecki SJ, Veir J. Effects of
a single dose of an intranasal feline herpesvirus 1, calicivirus,
and panleukopenia vaccine on clinical signs and virus shedding
after challenge with virulent feline herpesvirus 1. *J Fel. Med. Surg*
2006;8:158-163.

Ledwith, B.J., Manam, S., Troilo, P.J., Barnum, A.B., Pauley, C.J., Griffiths,
T.G. 2nd, Harper, L.B., Beare, C.M., Bagdon, W.J., and Nichols,
W.W. Plasmid DNA vaccines: Investigation of integration into host
cellular DNA following intramuscular injection in mice. *Intervirology*
2000, 43(4-6), 258-72.

Martin, T., Parker, S.E., Hedstrom, R., Le T., Hoffman, S.L., Norman, J.,
Hobart, P., and Lew, D.. Plasmid DNA malaria vaccine: the potential
for genomic integration after intramuscular injection. *Hum Gene Ther.*
1999, 10(5), 759-68.

Meeusen, E.N.T., Walker J., Peters A., Pastoret P-P., and Jungersen G.
2007. Current status of veterinary vaccines. *Clin. Microbiol. Rev* 20:
489-510.

O'Byrne, K.J., and Dalgleish, A.G. Chronic immune activation and
inflammation as the cause of malignancy. *British Journal of Cancer.*
2001 Aug 17;85(4):473-83.

Olson, M. E., D.W. Morck,, and H. Ceri. 1997. Preliminary data on the efficacy of a Giardia vaccine in puppies. *Can. Vet. J.* 38:777-779

Pashine, A., N., M. Valiante, and J. B Ulmer. 2005. Targeting the innate immune response with improved vaccine adjuvants. *Nat. Med.* 11:S63-S68.

Paul, M.A., Appel, M,J., Barrett, R., Carmichael, L.E., Childers, H., Cotter, S., Davidson, A., Ford, R., Keil, D., Lappin, M., Schultz, R.D., Thacker, E., Trumpeter, E., Welborn, L. Report of the American Animal Hospital Association (AAHA) *Canine Vaccine Task Force: 2003 Canine Vaccine Guidelines, Recommendations, and Supporting Literature*: http://www.britfeld.com/health/canine_vaccine_guidelines.pdf

Pulendran, B., and R Ahmed. 2006. Translating innate immunity into immunological memory: implications for vaccine development. *Cell* 124:849-863.

Robbins, S. C., M. D. Jelinski, and R. L. Stotish. 2004. Assessment of the immunological and biological efficacy of two different doses of a recombinant GnRH vaccine in domestic male and female cats (*Felis catus*). *J. Reprod. Immunol.* 64:107-119.

Rupprecht, C. E., C. A. Hanlon, and D. Slate. 2004. Oral vaccination of wildlife against rabies: opportunities and challenges in prevention and control. *Dev. Biol.* (Basel) 119:173-184.

Schetters, T. 2005. Vaccination against canine babesiosis. Trends Parasitol. 21:179-184

Schultz, R.D., R.B. Ford, J. Olsen, and F. Scott. 2002. Titer testing and vaccination: a new look at traditional practices. *Vet Med* 97: 1-13 (insert).

Schultz, R.D., Duration of immunity of canine and feline vaccines: a review. *Vet Microbiol* 2006, 117:75-79.

Smith, G.R. and S. Missailidis.2004. Cancer, inflammation, and the AT1 and AT2 receptors. *Journal of Inflammation*, 1:3.

Torch, W.S. 1982. Diptheria-pertussis-tetanus (DPT) immunizations: a potential cause of the sudden infant death syndrome (SIDS) *Neurology* 32-4 A169 abstract.

Traavik, T. An Orphan in Science: Environmental Risks of genetically Engineered Vaccines. *Research report No.1999-5* Directorate for Nature Management. Norway. www.naturforvaltning.no

United States Department of Agriculture (USDA), Center for Veterinary Biologics Notice Draft No. 327 on the subject of "Studies to Support Label Claims of Duration of Immunity:

http://www.aphis.usda.gov/animal_health/vet_biologics/
publications/Noticedraft327.pdf

Vilchez, R.A. et al 2002. Association between simian virus 40 and non-Hodgekin lymphoma *Lancet* Mar 9; 359(9309):817-823.

Villarreal, L.P. 2004. *Viruses and the Evolution of Life*. Washington DC, ASM Press.

World Small Animal Veterinary Association *Dog and Cat Vaccination Guidelines*: http://www.wsava.org/PDF/Misc/VGG_09_2007.pdf

CHAPTER 14

Note

(1) For more details see www.twobitdog.com/DrFox/ and OIE/world Organization for Animal Health, Manual of Diagnostic tests and Vaccines for Terrestrial Mammals, (2008). www.oieint/eng/normes/mmanual/A_00099.htm)

References

Appel, M., Bistner, S.I., Menegus, M., et al.(1973) Pathogenicity of low-virulence strains of two canine adenovirus types. *Am J Vey Res* 34, 543-550.

Beck, M.A. (2000) Nutritionally induced oxidative stress: effect on viral disease. Amer. J. Clinical Nutr 71, 1676S-1679s.

Bell, C.R., Scott, P., Sargison, D.J., et al (2010) Idiopathic neonatal pancytopenia in a Scottish beef herd.*Veterinary Record* 167, 938-940.

Botsch,V., Kuchenhoff, H.,.Hartmann, K. et al.(2009) Retrospective study of 871 dogs with thrombocytopenia. *Veterinary Record* 164,647-651.

Chan, V. (2006) Use of genetically modified viruses and genetically engineered virus-vector vaccines; Environmental effects. *J. Toxicology and Environmental Health Part A*. 69, 1971-1977.

Lassen, J.B., (1996) Childhood Immunisation and Diabetes Mellitus. *New Zealand M.J.*, 109, 195.

Cornwell, H.J., Thompson, H., McCandlish, I.A.P., et al (1988) Encephalitis in dogs associated with a batch of canine distemper (Rockborn) vaccine. *Veterinary Record*, 112, 54-59.

Dodds, W.J. (2001). Vaccination protocols for dogs predisposed to vaccine reactions. *J Am Animal Hosp Assoc* 38, 1-4.

Duval, D. &.Giger, U. (1996). Vaccine-Associated Immune-Mediated Hemolytic Anemia in the Dog, *Journal of Veterinary Internal Medicine* 10,290-295.

Fehiner-Gardiner, C., Nadin-Davis, S., Armstrong, J. et al (2008). ERA vaccine-derived cases of rabies in wildlife and domestic animals in Ontario, Canada, 1989-2004. *J. Wildlife Dis*, 44,71-85.

Fox, M.W. (2006) Principles of veterinary bioethics. *J Am Vet Med Assoc* 229, 666-667. See also FOX, M.W. *Bringing life to ethics: global bioethics for a humane society*. Albany NY: State University of New York Press,2001.

Goggs, R.,. Boag, A.K., & Chan, D.L., (2008) Concurrent immune-mediated haemolytic anaemia and severe thrombocytopenia in 21 dogs. *Veterinary Record* 163,323-327.

Hardin G.(1977) *The limits of altruism: an ecologists view of survival*. Bloomington: Indiana University Press.

Hogenesch, H., Azcona-Olivera, J. & Scott-Moncrieff, C. (1999). Vaccine-induced autoimmunity in the dog. *Adv Vet Med*. 41,733-747.

Kamal, S.A, (2009) Pathological studies of postvaccinal reactions of Rift Valley fever in goats. *Virol J*. 6, 94-103.

Lappin, M.R., Basaraba R.J., Jensen W.A. (2006) Interstitial nephritis in cats inoculated with Crandell Rees feline kidney cell lysates. *J. Feline Med. Surg*. 8,353-356.

Meeusen, E.N.T., Walker, J., Peters A. et al. (2007) Current status of veterinary vaccines. *Clin Microbiol Rev* 20, 489-510.

Iyazawa, T, Rokuseke, E Yoshikawa, R., Matthew, G. et al. (2010) Isolation of an Infectious Endogenous Retrovirus in a Proportion of Live Attenuated Vaccines for Pets. *J. Virol*. 84,3690-3694.

Montinari, M.G., Favoino, B., & Roberto, A. (1996) Role of immunogenetics in post-vaccine diseases of the central nervous system. *Mediterranean J. Surg & Med*. 4, 65-71.

Orbach, H., Agmon Levin, N., & Zandman Goddard, G. (2010) Vaccines and autoimmune diseases of the adult. *Discovery Med* 9, 90-97.

O'Toole, D.O.,& Campen H.Van. (2010) Abortifacient vaccines and bovine herpes virus1. *J Am Vet Med Assoc* 237. 259-260.

Pickles, K.J., Berger, J., Davies, R. et al (2011) use of gonadotrophin-releasing hormone vaccine in headshaking horses. *Veterinary Record* 168, 19.

Potter V.R. (1971) *Bioethics: bridge to the future*. Englewood Cliffs, NJ: Prentice Hall.

Scott-Moncrieff, J.C., Azcona-Olivera, J., Glickman, N.W. et al. (2002) Evaluation of antithyroglobulin antibodies after routine vaccination in pet and research dogs. *J Am Vet Med Assoc* 221, 515-521.

Shiel, R.E., Mooney, C.T., Brennan, S.F., Nolan, C. M. et al. (2010) Clinical and clinicopathological features of non-suppurative meningioencephalitis in young greyhounds in Ireland. *Veterinary Record* 167, 333-337

Smith, G.R., & Missailidis, S.(2004) Cancer, inflammation, and the AT1 and AT2 receptors. *J. Inflammation*, 1,3.

Spickler, A.R., & Roth, J.A. (2003) Adjuvants in veterinary vaccines: modes of action and adverse effects. *J Vet Inter Med*, 17, 273-281.

Taguchi, M., Namikawa, K., Mauruo, T. et al. (2010) Antibodies to parvovirus, distemper virus and adenovirus conferred to household dogs using commercial combination vaccines containing Leptospira bacterin. *Veterinary Record* 167, 931-934.

Traavik, T. (1999) An Orphan in Science: Environmental Risks of Genetically Engineered Vaccines. *Research Report No.1999-5* Directorate for Nature Management. Norway. www.naturforvaltning. no

Vilchez, R.A., Madden, C.R., Kozinetz, C.A. et al (2002) Association between simianvirus 40 and non-Hodgkin lymphoma. *Lancet* 9,359-817.

Additional References & Resources

Alexander, A. N., M. K. Huelsmeyer, A. Mitzey, et al (2006). Development of an allogeneic whole-cell tumor vaccine expressing xenogenic gp100 and its implementation in a phase II clinical trial in canine patients with malignant melanoma. Cancer Immunol. Immunother. 55:433-442.

American Veterinary Medical Association letter, re Center for Veterinary Biologics Notice Draft No. 327: Studies to Support Label Claims of Duration of Immunity dated October 27 2008: http://www.avma.org/advocacy/federal/regulatory/practice_ issues/vaccines/duration_of_immunity_ltr.pdf

Azad, N., and Y. Rojanasakul. (2006). Vaccine delivery—current trends and future. Curr. Drug Deliv. 3:137-146

Bergman, P.J., McKnight, J., Novosad, A., et al (2003) Long-term survival of dogs with advanced malignant melanoma after DNA vaccination with xenogeneic human tyrosinase: a phase I trial. Clin Cancer Res. 9(4), 1284-90.

Crawford, C. 2002. The Current Status of Canine Vaccinations: Are We Vaccinating Dogs With Too Many vaccines Too Often? Dog Owners and Breeders Symposium, University of Florida CVM.

Day, M.J., Horzinek, M.C.,& Schultz, R.D.(2007) Guidelines for the Vaccination of Dogs and Cats, compiled by the Vaccination

Guidelines Group (VGG) of the World Small Animal Veterinary Association (WSAVA). Journal of Small Animal Practice .
48 (9), 528-541: http://www.wsava.org/PDF/Misc/VGG_09_2007.pdf

Delves, P. J., T. Lund, & I. M. Roitt. (2002). Antifertility vaccines. Trends Immunol. 23:213-219.

de Vries, J.,& Meier, P., and Wackernagel, W. 2004. Microbial horizontal gene transfer and the DNA release from transgenic crop plants. Plant and Soil, 266: 91-104.

England, J. (2008). New Vaccine Technologies: Destined for Cattle Vaccines, CVC Proceedings. August 1st.

Frick, O.L., & D. L. Brooks. (1983) Immunoglobilin E antibodies in pollen-augmented in dogs by virus vaccines. Am. J. Vet Res. 44: 440-445.

Friedrich, F. et al (1996). Temporal association between the isolation of Sabin-related poliovirus vaccine strains and the Guillan-Barre syndrome Rev Inst Med Trop. Sao Paulo, Jan-Feb; 38(1):55-8.

Hardham, J., M. Reed, J. Wong, et al (2005). Evaluation of a monovalent companion animal periodontal disease vaccine in an experimental mouse periodontitis model. Vaccine 23:3148-3156.

Isaguliants, M.G., Iakimtchouk, K., Petrakova, N.V., et al (2004) Gene immunization may induce secondary antibodies reacting with DNA. Vaccine 2004, 22(11-12),1576-85.

Kirpensteijn, J.(2006) Feline injection site-associated sarcoma: Is it a reason to critically evaluate our vaccination policies? Vet Microbiol. 117: 59-65.

Kowalczyk, D. & Ertl H. (1999) Immune response to DNA vaccines. CMLS Cell. Mol. Life Sci. 55, 751-70.

Kuiken, T., G. Rimmelzwaan, D. van Riel, et al. (2004) Avian H5N1 influenza in cats. Science 306:241.

Lappin, M.R., Sebring RW, Porter M, et al. (2006) Effects of a single dose of an intranasal feline herpesvirus 1, calicivirus, and panleukopenia vaccine on clinical signs and virus shedding after challenge with virulent feline herpesvirus 1. J Fel. Med. Surg 8:158-163.

Ledwith, B.J., Manam, S., Troilo, P.J., et al. (2000) Plasmid DNA vaccines: Investigation of integration into host cellular DNA following intramuscular injection in mice. Intervirology 43(4-6), 258-72.

Martin, T., Parker, S.E., Hedstrom, R., Le T., et al. (1999) Plasmid DNA malaria vaccine: the potential for genomic integration after intramuscular injection. Hum Gene Ther. 10(5), 759-68.

O'Byrne, K.J., & Dalgleish, A.G.(2001) Chronic immune activation and inflammation as the cause of malignancy. British Journal of

Cancer.;85(4):473-83.

Olson, M. E., D.W. Morck, & H. Ceri. (1997) Preliminary data on the efficacy of a Giardia vaccine in puppies. Can. Vet. J. 38:777-779

Pashine, A., N., M. Valiante,& J. B Ulmer. (2005)Targeting the innate immune response with improved vaccine adjuvants. Nat. Med. 11:S63-S68.

Paul, M.A., Appel, M,J., Barrett, et al (2003) Report of the American Animal Hospital Association (AAHA) Canine Vaccine Task Force: 2003 Canine Vaccine Guidelines, Recommendations, and Supporting Literature: http://www.britfeld.com/health/canine_vaccine_guidelines.pdf

Pulendran, B., & R Ahmed. (2006). Translating innate immunity into immunological memory: implications for vaccine development. Cell 124:849-863.

Robbins, S. C., M. D. Jelinski, & R. L. Stotish. (2004) Assessment of the immunological and biological efficacy of two different doses of a recombinant GnRH vaccine in domestic male and female cats (Felis catus). J. Reprod. Immunol. 64:107-119.

Rupprecht, C. E., C. A. Hanlon, & D. Slate. (2004) Oral vaccination of wildlife against rabies: opportunities and challenges in prevention and control. Dev. Biol. (Basel) 119:173-184.

Schetters, T. (2005) Vaccination against canine babesiosis. Trends Parasitol. 21:179-184.

Schultz, R.D., R.B. Ford, J. Olsen ET AL and F. Scott. (2002) Titer testing and vaccination: a new look at traditional practices. *Vet Med* 97: 1-13 (insert).

Schultz, R.D. (2006) Duration of immunity of canine and feline vaccines: a review. Vet Microbiol 2006, 117:75-79.

Torch, W.S. (1982) Diptheria-pertussis-tetanus (DPT) immunizations: a potential cause of the sudden infant death syndrome (SIDS) Neurology 32-4 A169 abstract.

United States Department of Agriculture (USDA), Center for Veterinary Biologics Notice Draft No. 327 on the subject of "Studies to Support Label Claims of Duration of Immunity: http://www.aphis.usda.gov/animal_health/vet_biologics/ publications/Noticedraft327.pdf

Villarreal, L.P. (2004) Viruses and the Evolution of Life. Washington DC, ASM Press.

World Small Animal Veterinary Association Dog and Cat Vaccination Guidelines: http://www.wsava.org/PDF/Misc/VGG_09_2007.pdf

CHAPTER **15**

For more details on this modern food crisis and its adverse effects on companion animals, see *Not Fit For a Dog: The Truth About Manufactured Dog And Cat Food* by veterinarians Drs. M.W. Fox, E. Hodgkins, and M. E. Smart, published in 2008 by Quill Driver Books, Sanger, CA.

References & End Notes

Organically certified foods of both animal and plant origin contain more essential nutrients, notably antioxidants, than conventionally grown produce, and of course cause less environmental harms and are pesticide free. For documentation, see Cooper J, Leifert C, and Niggily U, (eds) *Handbook of Organic Food Safety and Quality*. Cambridge, UK, Woodhead Publ. Inc. 2007. For evidence that organic farming methods can feed the hungry world, see Badgley C, et al, Organic agriculture and the global food supply. *Renewable Agriculture and Food Systems*, 22:86-108, 2007.

Campbell, T.C, *The China Study*: The most comprehensive study of nutrition conducted, and the startling implication for diet, weight-loss and long-term health. Dallas TX Bell Bella Books, 2005.

Fox, M.W. *Bringing Life to Ethics: Global Bioethics for a Humane Society*. Albany, NY. State University of New York Press, 2001.

News and Reports. Rats reveal risks of 'junk food' during pregnancy. *The Veterinary Record*, Aug 18, p 215, 2007.

Steinfeld, H, P. Gerber P, Wassenaer T, Castel V, Rosales M, and de Haan C, *Livestock's Long Shadow: Environmental Issues and Options*. United Nation's Food and Agriculture Organization, Washington, DC, 2004.

CHAPTER **17**

Michael W. Fox, *The Whistling Hunters: Studies of the Asiatic Wild Dog, Cuon alpinus*. Albany NY. State University of New York Press, 1984.

CHAPTER **18**

1. Day, M.J. One health: the small animal dimension. *Veterinary Record* 2010; 167: 847-850.
2. Chan, V. Use of genetically modified viruses and genetically engineered virus-vector vaccines; Environmental effects. *J. Toxicology and*

Environmental Health Part A.2006; **69:**1971-1977.

3. Dodds, W.J. Vaccination protocols for dogs predisposed to vaccine reactions. *J Am Animal Hosp Assoc* 2001; 38 1-4.

4. Orbach, H., Levin N. Zandman Goddard G. Vaccines and autoimmune diseases of the adult. *Discovery Med* 2010; 9: 90-97.

5. Schwabe, C.W. *Cattle, priests and progress in medicine.* Minneapolis MN: University of Minnesota Press, 1978.

6. Fox, M.W. *Concepts in ethology: animal and human behavior.* Minneapolis MN: University of Minnesota Press, 1974.

7. Fox, M.W. Veterinarians and animal rights. *California Veterinarian* 1983;1:15-16 & 98.

8. Nielsen, N.O. Ecosystem health and veterinary medicine. *Can Vet J* 1992;33:23-26.

9. Vanleeuwen, J.A., Nielsen, N.O. and Waltner-Toews D. Ecosystem health: an essential filed for veterinary medicine. *J Am Vet Med Assoc* 1998;212: 53-57.

10. Fox, M.W. Veterinary bioethics: ecoveterinary and ethnoveterinary perspectives. *Vet Res Commun* 1995; 19: 9-15.

11. Smith, J.M. *Genetic roulette: the documented health risks of genetically engineered foods.* Fairfield Iowa Yes! Books 2007.

12. Schweitzer, A. *Out of my life and thought: an autobiography.* New York: Holt, Rinehart and Winston, p.158-9, 1961.

13. de Montaudouin, Maya. Personal communication. See also her book: M. Montaudouin MXM *Man out of Mutant: a Personal Quest for a Creed to Live By.* Columbus, N.C: Good Earth Publications.1996.

14. Potter, V.R. *Bioethics: Bridge to the future.* Englewood Cliffs: Prentice Hall, 1971.

15. Fox, M.W. Principles of veterinary bioethics. *J Am Vet Med Assoc* 2006; 229: 666-667. See also Fox MW. *Bringing life to ethics: global bioethics for a humane society.* Albany NY: State University of New York Press,2001.

16. Hardin, G. *The Limits of Altruism: An Ecologists View of Survival.* Bloomington: Indiana University Press, 1977.

17. News. Data show volume of antimicrobials sold. *J Am Vet Med Assoc* 2011; 238:273.

18. Elliott, C. *White Coat, Black Hat: Adventures on the Dark Side of Medicine.* Boston: Beacon Press, 2011.

ABOUT THE AUTHOR

MICHAEL W. FOX was born and educated in the UK, earning his veterinary degree on a Derbyshire County Exhibition Scholarship studying at the Royal Veterinary College, London, from where he graduated in 1962, with honors in pathology and animal husbandry. He was awarded the gold medal and Fellowship of the Veterinary Medical Association by the Royal Veterinary College for his research report on Diseases of the Sheep-dog in Relation to Management and Nutrition. His subsequent research into animal behavior and development in the U.S. resulted in a dissertation entitled Integrative Development of the Brain and Behavior in the Dog (published in 1971 by the University of Chicago Press), that earned a Ph.D. in Medicine from London University in 1967.

After receiving the Outstanding Teacher Faculty Award from the Alumni at Washington University, St Louis, Missouri, where he continued behavioral and developmental studies in dogs, cats, wolves, coyotes, foxes, and other related canids, for which he earned a D.Sc. in animal behavior/ethology from London University in 1976, he chose to focus on advocating animal protection, rights and environmental conservation, and in continuing his avocation as a teacher and public speaker. Between 1967 and 2003 he served in various positions with the Humane Society of the United States, including Scientific Director and Vice President for Bioethics and Sustainable Agriculture. During this time he was a regular guest on Johnny Carson's Tonight Show, and published two bestselling books, *Understanding Your Dog*, and *Understanding Your Cat*. He was chairman of the National Academy of Science (NAS) Committee on Applied Animal Ethology, and served on the National Academy of Science's Committee on Laboratory Animal Care and Standards for Dogs and Cats. He was also a member of the Council for Agriculture, Science and Technology Task Force on Farm Animal Welfare, and was an advisor to the National Organics Standards Board on farm animal health, welfare and humane sustainable agriculture.

He has authored and edited over 40 books for adults and children, and writes the nationally syndicated newspaper column, *Animal Doctor* (with United Features Syndicate, NY). His regular monthly animal column in

McCall's magazine was the longest running column on animals in a U.S. magazine. Featured in Marquis' *Who's Who in America*, *Who's Who in Science and Technology*, and *Who's Who in the World*, Dr. Fox is a widely recognized author, consultant, and lecturer: On animal awareness, emotions, rights, and well-being; on human- nonhuman relationships and rights philosophy; and, on bioethics, biotechnology, humane, sustainable agriculture, and holistic health. His long-held basic premise—that human health and well being are inseparable from animal health and welfare and environmental protection and conservation—is now gaining international recognition as a bioethical imperative and prerequisite for a viable future.

He is a member of the British Veterinary Association, the American Holistic Veterinary Medical Association and an Honor Roll Member of the American Veterinary Medical Association.

COLOPHON
Type Face: Baskerville 11/14
Display Face: Arial 14/14
Design: M.W. Fox & A.E. Wittbecker
Photographs & graphics: M.W. Fox
Editing & Formatting: A. E. Wittbecker
Software: Word, Photoshop, Indesign
Hardware: Mac G5, HP 3310